NISTIR 7743

Usability in Health IT: Technical Strategy, Research, and Implementation
Summary of Workshop

I0438646

Janice (Ginny) Redish

Redish & Associates, Inc.

Svetlana Z. Lowry
Information Access Division
Information Technology Laboratory

National Institute of Standards and Technology

November 2010

U.S. Department of Commerce

Gary Locke, Secretary

National Institute of Standards and Technology

Patrick D. Gallagher, Director

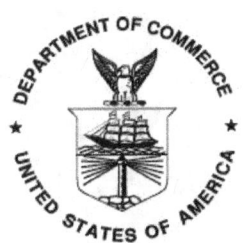

Usability in Health IT: Technical Strategy, Research, and Implementation

Summary of Workshop
July 13, 2010
National Institute of Standards and Technology
Gaithersburg, MD 20899

Workshop Coordinators

Matthew Quinn
Agency for Healthcare Research and Quality
U.S. Department of Health and Human Services
540 Gaither Road
Rockville, MD 20851

Svetlana Lowry
National Institute of Standards and Technology
U.S. Department of Commerce
1 Bureau Drive
Gaithersburg, MD 20899

Sachin Jain
Charles Friedman
Office of the National Coordinator for Health Information Technology
U.S. Department of Health and Human Services
200 Independence Avenue S.W.
Suite 729-D
Washington, D.C. 20201

Table of Contents

Executive Summary

On July 13, 2010, 27 roundtable discussion participants and more than 100 other attendees gathered at the National Institute of Standards and Technology (NIST) for a full-day workshop on *Usability in Health IT: Technical Strategy, Research, and Implementation.* The workshop brought together people from the federal government, the electronic health record (EHR) and health information technology industries, healthcare providers, and universities to share current activities and consider technical strategies and tactics for improving the usability and accessibility of EHRs.

Usability is defined by international standards as "the extent to which a product can be used by specified users to achieve specified goals with effectiveness, efficiency, and satisfaction in a specified context of use." Accessibility is the need to make sure any IT system works for all the people who must use it.

Usability and accessibility are critical because, to improve care and outcomes, information systems must work well for the people who use them. Care providers ultimately use and act on the information provided through EHRs. No matter the functionality provided, an information system is for naught if clinicians and others cannot find what they need, understand what they find, and use the technology effectively, efficiently, safely, and with satisfaction.

EHRs are of considerable interest and importance now because the American Recovery and Reinvestment Act (ARRA), enacted by Congress in February 2009, allocates considerable funding to promote the meaningful use of EHRs in the United States. Usability and accessibility, many believe, are critical to increasing adoption and meaningful use.

The workshop was sponsored by the Agency for Healthcare Quality and Research (AHRQ), the National Institute of Standards and Technology (NIST), and the Office of the National Coordinator for Health Information Technology (ONC). AHRQ and ONC are both part of the U.S. Department of Health and Human Services (HHS).

In a day that included several short presentations and an open discussion among the roundtable participants and with the audience, the following key points emerged:

- Usability is critical to adoption and meaningful use.

- Accessibility is also critical.

- Usability is often misunderstood.

- Education about usability and accessibility is needed now by developers, vendors, buyers, and users.

- We know a lot about some aspects of usability.

- Some resources exist that can help us start to provide guidance now.

- Usability can be measured both qualitatively and quantitatively.

- Many factors impact usability, including workflow, time pressure, physical environment, social environment, organizational policies of use, and personal attributes of users – age, language, literacy, personal health, stress, disabilities.

- Standardization can support usability.

- Usability and research on usability must be continuous, ongoing.

- Training is an issue that must be considered. Some speakers argued for systems that are simple because health care professionals cannot take the time to be trained – and physicians who attend in several hospitals may work with several different systems. Other speakers argued that an EHR will always be inherently too complex – even if well-designed for usability – to be usable without training.

- How to train future health care professionals so they are comfortable with EHRs early in their careers is also an issue that must be considered.

Participants and audience members also gave the government agencies present at least 28 recommendations for further action. You will find these listed on pages 14 – 15 of the report.

The report that follows includes:

- an overview;

- a summary of the key points made during the day with a list of recommendations that came out of the open discussion;

- summaries of each speaker's presentation;

- a person-by-person summary of each contribution to the open discussion;

- 6 appendices.

1. Introduction

Twenty-seven roundtable discussion participants and more than 100 other attendees gathered on July 13, 2010, at the National Institute of Standards and Technology (NIST), for a full-day workshop on *Usability in Health IT: Technical Strategy, Research, and Implementation*. The workshop brought together people from the federal government, the EHR and technology industries, healthcare providers, and universities to share current activities and consider technical strategies and tactics for improving the usability and accessibility of electronic health records (EHRs).

Workshop Objectives

The workshop objectives were to

- Establish an immediate set of actions in usability and accessibility to inform the national initiative to drive adoption and meaningful use of EHRs

- Develop a strategic approach to measuring and assessing the usability and accessibility of EHRs

- Inspire follow-on activities in both the public and private sectors

Background

The American Recovery and Reinvestment Act (ARRA), enacted by Congress in February 2009, allocates considerable funding to promote the meaningful use of EHRs in the United States. This funding is based on the belief that increased use of health IT could address many persistent problems in the quality of healthcare as well as help control spiraling costs.

To promote adoption and use, the Department of Health and Human Services (HHS) will soon be offering incentives for doctors and hospitals to use information technology and integrate it in a meaningful way into their healthcare delivery processes.

NIST's role

The National Institute of Standards and Technology (NIST) is playing a key role in many health IT initiatives, including accessibility, certification, interoperability, privacy, security, testing, and usability.

This workshop and NIST's several initiatives in health IT are in keeping with NIST's mission to promote U.S. innovation and industrial competitiveness by advancing measurement science, standards, and technology in ways that enhance economic security and improve our quality of life. They focus directly on NIST's three core competencies:

- Measurement science

- Rigorous traceability

- Development and use of standards

AHRQ's role

The mission of the Agency for Healthcare Research and Quality (AHRQ) is to improve the quality, safety, efficiency, and effectiveness of health care for all Americans. The promise of health IT in supporting this mission depends a great deal on how clinicians use health IT systems at the point of care. AHRQ has currently invested over $300 million dollars in health IT initiatives to promote the planning, implementation, and use of health IT.

Insight gained from work in usability has the capability of enhancing the value of past, present, and future AHRQ investments in health IT and provides leadership in an area not currently being prioritized or effectively addressed by the private sector. AHRQ's work in usability supports key long and short term program goals for the health IT portfolio.

ONC's role

The Office of the National Coordinator for Health Information Technology (ONC) is the principal Federal entity charged with coordinating nationwide efforts to implement and use the most advanced health information technology and the electronic exchange of health information. The position of National Coordinator was created in 2004, through an Executive Order, and legislatively mandated in the Health Information Technology for Economic and Clinical Health Act of 2009 (HITECH).

Both AHRQ and ONC are part of the U.S. Department of Health and Human Services (HHS).

This workshop focused on usability and accessibility

The July 13, 2010, workshop focused on usability and accessibility of health information technology, especially electronic health records (EHRs).

Usability (as defined by ISO 9241, Part 11) is "the extent to which a product can be used by specified users to achieve specified goals with effectiveness, efficiency, and satisfaction in a specified context of use."

Accessibility is the need to make sure any IT system works for all the people who must use it. (See www.webaim.org.)

Usability and accessibility are critical because people are a very important (and complex and unpredictable) part of any IT system. They are the ones that ultimately make use of and act on the information being provided. Information systems would have no reason to exist if it were not for human users. No matter what functionality is provided in an IT system, that functionality is for naught if people cannot find what they need, understand what they find, and use the technology effectively, efficiently, safely, and with satisfaction.

Structure of the Day

The day included:

- welcoming remarks;
- a keynote address;
- four sessions of short talks (7 minutes each);
- question and answer (Q&A) among the panel and with the audience after each session;
- open discussion on recommendations and next steps.

Welcoming remarks

Two of the workshop sponsors started the day with welcoming remarks:

- Ms. Cita M. Furlani, Director, Information Technology Laboratory, NIST; and
- Dr. Charles Friedman, Chief Scientific Officer, Office of the National Coordinator for Health Information Technology.

Keynote

The keynote address followed these opening remarks. In the keynote, Dr. Neil Patel, Associate Medical Director, Special Care Center, Atlantic City, NJ, described how EHRs have (and have not) worked for his highly-innovative, team-based, proactive medical practice.

Short talks

In the rest of the morning and early afternoon, we heard short talks (7 minutes each) from 26 speakers, divided into four panels. The panel topics were:

- Current State of EHRs and Need for Action
- Measuring and Reporting Usability
- "Points of Pain" – Addressing EHR User Disparities
- Defining Federal Strategy: ONC, NIST, AHRQ, and FDA Usability Collective Efforts

Each panel session ended with a short time for audience questions and responses from panel members. The talks had to be so short to accommodate the many experts who had important information to share. The audience questions and panel's responses after each session were extremely limited because the agenda called for a long time for open discussion in the afternoon.

Open discussion: Recommendations and next steps

For approximately two hours in the afternoon, the workshop was opened to general discussion among the panel members and with the audience.

The focus of this discussion was to generate recommendations and next steps for the technical strategy, research, and implementation of EHR usability and accessibility.

Structure of this Report

In Chapter 2, we summarize key points from the speakers' presentations, as well as recommendations for next steps from the discussion session.

In Chapter 3, we highlight the main points of each speaker's presentation and of the short question and answer sessions after each panel.

In Chapter 4, we report on the discussion that took place in the afternoon participatory session.

Several appendices give you details:

Appendix A	Final Agenda
Appendix B	List of Invited Workshop Participants
Appendix C	Speakers' Biographies
Appendix D	Presentation Summaries (abstracts of their talks as provided by the speakers)
Appendix E	Acronyms Used in the Report
Appendix F	References and Resources Mentioned by Speakers

All the speakers who used slides have allowed their slide sets to be posted on the NIST Web site. These slide sets are available all together with the final agenda as a single PDF file (25 MG) at: http://www.nist.gov/itl/upload/Final-Agenda-Usability-in-Health-IT-2.pdf.

A few presenters included their speaking notes with the slides. You can see these by clicking on the small call-out icon when it appears in the upper left corner of a slide.

2. Key Points and Recommendations That Emerged From the Workshop

Key Points

In their presentations, the workshop speakers made these key points:

Usability is critical to adoption and meaningful use

- Usability is critical to increasing adoption and meaningful use of EHRs.

- Poor usability is a barrier to adoption and meaningful use.

- Greater usability and interoperability will lead to wider adoption.

- Lack of usability in an EHR can cause not only frustration, non-use, and non-adoption. It can be harmful when medical errors occur because a user could not find or did not see relevant information.

- Both utility (usefulness, how well a system handles the work a user must do) and ease-of-use are part of usability.

Accessibility is also critical

- Accessibility is also critical for EHRs. EHRs must be usable to all, and people with special needs exist within all the relevant communities, including health professionals, patients, and administrators.

- Accessibility is related to and a companion to usability but is not identical to usability. We need usability for all, that is, accessibility.

- To achieve accessibility, we must have ways to make interfaces flexible. We cannot plan to have vendors build a separate interface for each individual. Rather, the interfaces must be adaptable so that individuals can change the interfaces to meet their needs.

- At least one project is under way to make that flexibility happen: The National Public Inclusive Infrastructure (NPII).

Usability is often misunderstood

- Among vendors and buyers (practitioners), usability is often equated only with user satisfaction. But usability is about effectiveness and efficiency as well as satisfaction. Usability is about helping clinicians get the right treatment to the right patient at the right time.

- However, perception is important; and systems also have to be convenient, pleasurable, and meaningful. People use systems that they like, that they feel comfortable with, that give them value without overloading them.

- Usability is also about helping people avoid errors and recovering easily from errors – building easy-to-follow paths that keep people from errors rather than relying on alerts which many experienced users tend to ignore.

We need education now

- Educating both vendors and buyers that usability is not just satisfaction but also (even more importantly) effectiveness and efficiency is critical.

- The timing of education, toolkits, guidance, frameworks, and further certification is going to be critical. Hospitals and clinicians are buying and upgrading now to take advantage of incentives. We cannot wait even two years to educate vendors and buyers about usability and accessibility. We need to give them at least some guidance now. Non-government groups are doing that (for example, HIMSS' new draft guide, *Selecting an EMR for Your Practice: Evaluating Usability*.)

- Audiences beyond vendors need education and guidance. In particular, the people who are customizing, configuring, and implementing systems need to be conscious of usability as they change systems.

We know a lot about some aspects of usability; we can provide (some) guidance now

- EHR developers do not have to start from scratch in creating guidelines for either accessibility or usability.

- Many resources already exist that provide relevant guidance on issues such as user interactions, cognitive load, screen design, message design, and so on. (See Appendix F for a list of the resources that were mentioned by different people in the workshop.)

Usability can be measured, but...

- Usability can be measured. Both qualitative and quantitative measures exist for usability. Each has its benefits. Qualitative measures give rich descriptions and help us see problems and potential solutions. Quantitative measures allow objective comparisons but do not give the rich data on sources of problems. Quantitative measures also require careful controls.

- A single usability score does not give enough information to help vendors or buyers.

- Many factors impact usability, including
  - workflow
  - time pressure
  - physical environment – lighting, room layout
  - social environment

   – organizational policies of use

   – personal attributes, such as age, language, literacy, personal health, stress, disabilities

Several speakers cautioned that EHR developers and vendors, EHR buyers, and usability testers have to be aware of these factors.

- Many people use EHRs (physicians, nurses, administrative staff, patients, etc.). How do we assure usability for all these user groups?

- Testing usability in a laboratory setting can reveal many problems, but will not be a true measure of actual usability. (A system that does poorly in a laboratory-based usability test will almost certainly do even more poorly in real use. However, a system that seems effective and efficient in a laboratory setting may fail in real use because of all the other factors listed above.)

Standardization can support usability

- Design standards would benefit both vendors and users. Speakers gave examples, such as standardizing date formats, and pointed to other industries with standardization, such as automobile design. We can all move from one car to another without a large learning curve. Speakers also pointed to resources on patterns and pattern language – a way that many software and web application vendors make products easy to learn by designing components in ways that are familiar to users.

- Patterns may be very useful as they have been in other domains. Many pattern libraries exist for software development.

Usability and research on usability must be continuous, ongoing

- Usability is a continuous process. It's not something we do once and assume the product is therefore usable forever after.

- Research on usability is also an ongoing endeavor. In other domains, even very well established ones like aerospace, human factors and usability research is funded continuously.

- Future: We should be talking not only about health *information* technology but also about health *improvement* technology. We have to come into the digital age and have common user interfaces for common EHR functions.

Training is an issue

- Training is going to be a big challenge. On the one hand, EHRs are complex systems. We cannot expect them to be "walk-up-and-use" like a kiosk. On the other hand, health care professionals want to spend their time caring for patients and not learning a new software tool. And certainly not learning three or four different EHR systems as can happen if a doctor practices at several hospitals.

- Speakers disagreed on how simple an EHR can be. Some called for great simplicity. Others likened an EHR to the complexity of a NASA control station or an airplane cockpit.

- We must consider not only how to train people on the job but also how to train future practitioners.

Tensions exist on some topics that will impact system development

- Tension exists between the desire for interoperability (an EHR works seamlessly with other systems, such as laboratory results, client registration and management, report writing, etc.) and vendors' desire to sell an entire suite (that is, their main EHR works only with their version of each of these other product types).

- Tension also exists in health IT (as in any other domain) between people's expectations (and often desires) that new software will follow their current patterns of work and using the software to help people get into more effective and efficient workflows.

- An important question to consider: How do we shift the paradigm from systems that are just documenting things as they are now (paper form becomes digital) to systems that help clinicians make faster, better decisions, that help clinicians deliver the right treatment to the right patient at the right time?

Recommendations to Government

Workshop participants and audience members contributed many recommendations to the government sponsors of the workshop.

- Provide leadership, as, for example, convening this workshop.

- Provide continuing research: Have a comprehensive research agenda on usability and accessibility in health IT. Fund it; carry it out; disseminate findings and lessons learned.

- Include usability and accessibility in meaningful use; promulgate the concept of *meaningful usability*.

- Hold hearings, involving all stakeholders including the disability community, on what meaningful usability and accessibility would look like.

- Elevate accessibility to be a top concern, at the same level as security, interoperability, and usability.

- Include accessibility in all activities: strategic plan, standards, certification, etc.

- Increase government staffing for health IT research and resources.

- Find out what other countries have done and what they have learned and make use of that knowledge.

- Create a framework for usability.

- Provide standards, guidelines, and best practices to vendors and to the user community.

- Disseminate information for educating vendors, buyers, customizers, etc. **now**, even if it is preliminary information – based on knowledge developed in other domains.

- Use social media to share information.

- Provide guidance to purchasers on how to put appropriate language into requests for proposals to vendors that would require vendors to differentiate offers on the basis of usability. (Both Dr. Lowry of NIST and Mr. Baquis of the U.S. Access Board said that this already exists for usability and for accessibility. So the issue may be one of making people aware of these resources and explaining why they would want to use them.)

- Develop standards, such as standard formats, data standards, standard keys and conventions – for example, where search comes on the screen.

- Develop, disseminate, and enforce standard vocabularies (like SNOMED CT) that would enable cross-system comparisons.

- Develop certification criteria and protocols.

- Decide on objective measures of usability.

- Set usability goals for systems; for example, a physician in a small medical practice will be able to get to a patient's laboratory results in xx seconds – and communicate these usability goals to vendors and the user community.

- Gather reliable comparative data on systems so buyers can look up, for example, average time to complete the same tasks in different systems – based on actual performance by real users.

- Focus on user- and task-based usability testing where actual users do actual tasks.

- Begin at the intersection of usability and safety.

- Research typical errors with EHRs, how many, how severe, about what, how users recover, what types of alerts and messages work and don't work.

- Focus on how systems handle data and errors (including potential errors – i.e., alerts).

- Refine reporting mechanisms for error events and help clinicians figure out what happened in an error situation and report it.

- Develop a formal process for capturing incidents, perhaps working from what the Department of Veterans Affairs has already developed.

- Push for interoperability, not only for components like lab results, but also for customer relationship management, email, chat, pictures, and more.

- Make systems and communications visual and do more research on how well specific types of visuals work in this domain for these audiences.

- Find ways to migrate workflow management technology into health IT.

3. Summary of Each Short Talk

In this chapter, we give the main points of each speaker's presentation. The chapter is organized chronologically, starting with the opening remarks.

Welcome Remarks and Keynote

We began the day with opening remarks from two of the workshop's sponsors, followed by a talk from a medical practitioner about the realities of using an EHR.

Opening remarks from NIST

Cita M. Furlani
Director, Information Technology Laboratory (ITL)
National Institute of Standards and Technology (NIST)

Ms. Furlani welcomed the workshop attendees to NIST. She explained how appropriate it is that the workshop was being held at NIST because the workshop topics (standards and measurement) are the central focus of NIST's mission. She invited attendees to take time in the day to visit the museum at NIST of the many contributions NIST makes to standards and measurement.

Furlani also emphasized the importance of both usability and accessibility. NIST has been involved in usability for more than a decade. Describing several activities within ITL, Ms. Furlani cited, in particular, ITL's work in voting. Scientists in ITL have developed standards for both usability and accessibility of voting systems, in support of the Help America Vote Act.

Opening remarks from the Office of the National Coordinator for Health Information Technology

Dr. Charles Friedman
Chief Scientific Office
Office of the National Coordinator for Health Information Technology (ONC)

Dr. Friedman also welcomed the workshop attendees, explaining that he brought greetings from the National Coordinator and others who could not be at the workshop because the final rule on meaningful use was being announced that same day.

Friedman brought together the topics of meaningful use and usability when he declared that "meaningful use requires usability." He went on to say, "Usability of EHR systems is absolutely critical to get the nation's physicians to effectively use that software." And he said further, "Uneven or poor usability, to the extent that it exists, is a barrier to health IT adoption and must be overcome."

As Friedman pointed out, usability is a continuous, ongoing process. It's not just something we do once and assume is there, forever.

He said that we must not expect users to think like the machines, but rather that "machines that think like users will promote adoption."

He also brought out one of the main themes of the day: that usability is a science with measurement methods and data, but many in the vendor and practitioner communities are not as aware of that as they need to be. We must make the case to them. ONC wants usability standards to inform clinicians' purchasing decisions and, thus, improve systems over time.

Keynote: Why are electronic health records hard to use?
The good, the bad, and the ugly: Implementing an electronic health record in an innovative medical home practice

Neil Patel, M.D.
Associate Medical Director
Special Care Center
Atlantic City, NJ

Dr. Patel spoke about his experience as a family practitioner using an EHR in a very innovative, team-based, proactive medical setting. His practice provides medical care to members of the Hotel Workers' Union. As he explained, his patients are low-wage workers doing heavy physical work. Most are limited-English-speakers, often with low literacy in any language.

Trying to stem the rising cost of health care, Patel and his team focus on the five to ten percent of patients who have so many and multiple health problems that they account for about 65 percent of the union's health care costs. Working as a team and using an EHR, Patel's group is proactive in getting their patients to come to the Special Care Center, to make sure these patients get and take their medications, start – and continue – appropriate physical exercise, stop smoking, and so on.

The team-based, pro-active approach has been very successful. Compared to other approaches, the Special Care Center has very high rates of success in having patients stop smoking, lower their blood pressure, and control cholesterol.

Of particular interest for the workshop were the ways in which the EHR that Patel's group uses supports (and does not support) this innovative practice.

Good

Benefits of using the EHR include

- Legibility. Doctors' handwriting is often difficult to read.

- Many users. All team members can put data in and view data. Different people can be looking at the chart in different rooms at the same time. The chart doesn't get lost.

- Automating tasks. For example, the pharmacy gets the prescription automatically. Prescriptions are often ready for patients by the time they get downstairs to the pharmacy.

- Enhancing safety. Especially for making sure that prescriptions are filled correctly and the team knows all medications the patient is taking.

Bad

However, the EHR fails the practice in some ways:

- Errors creep into the medication list.

- When they find a problem, they can't fix it. They need a programmer to understand the need, figure out how to fix it, and program the fix.

- The software crashes, and when it does, they have no records to work from.

- Lab results are not integrated into the system.

- The decision-support system is overdone. Clinical warnings and alerts come so frequently and many are so obvious that doctors ignore them – potentially ignoring a critical warning that was not obvious and did need attention.

Ugly

Patel described ways in which the EHR that his practice uses makes work particularly challenging for their innovative practice. The EHR

- assumes a single physician practice; it does not support working as a team

- does not support pro-active medicine of the sort that Patel's group practices – where they regularly contact their patients and follow-up with them rather than waiting for the patient to contact the doctor

- does not have a patient registration system

- can't give integrative reports to help manage the practice. For example, it can't search the records to show which patients have stopped smoking.

- is basically an electronic copy of the old paper forms

In conclusion, Patel suggested that instead of asking "Why are electronic health records hard to use?" we might ask two other questions:

- What are electronic records really designed to do?

- How can we rethink our design specifications to make EHRs more usable?

For more on the topic of Patel's talk, see Fernandopulle and Patel, 2010.

Panel 1: Current State of EHRs and Need for Action

In the first session of short talks, we heard from six speakers with a variety of perspectives on the current state of EHRs and the need for action.

Meaningful use: Meaning more? Or meaning less? Defining and defying sub-clinical HIT

Ross Koppel, Ph.D.
Professor, Department of Sociology
University of Pennsylvania

Dr. Koppel, a sociologist, has been involved in reviewing many EHRs. In this talk, he compared the pre-HITECH situation with the new situation, in which we have the Health Information Technology for Economic and Clinical Health Act of 2009 (HITECH), NIST's involvement, the meaningful use rule, usability testing, and certification of EHRs.

While saying that "HITECH is so much better than the previous system," Koppel also pointed out tensions that still exist, such as:

- Between bench testing and in-situ testing

- Between making products interoperable and vendors' desire to sell an entire suite of products

On bench testing versus in-situ testing, Koppel pointed out that Certification Commission for Health Information Technology (CCHIT) testing involves committees watching vendors demonstrate their products. It does not exercise those products in real settings. Giving credit to the CCHIT judges' very hard work, Koppel also expressed concern about systems that pass CCHIT certification even when, as in the example he cited, several engineers took eight hours to input a complex order. As Koppel said, doctors cannot spend that amount of time with an EHR on one order, even if it is a complex order.

Not having in-situ testing allows vendors to argue that their software is fine and that all the problems are introduced in implementation.

On interoperability and usability, Koppel pointed out that, in the past, neither was a factor in most discussions of adoption or reviews of products. He cited a 2009 paper by Jha, DesRoches, Campbell, et al. on what hospitals perceived as facilitators of EHR adoption. That study included no questions – and, therefore, no findings – on usability or interoperability.

Both of these tensions are important because adoption depends on the systems working for practitioners in the realistic conditions of their practice. Koppel argued that greater usability and interoperability will lead to wider adoption, which is the goal of HITECH.

Best practices in usability and information design of electronic health records

Kristen Werner, M.H.S.A.
Senior Analyst, Health Information and Technology Strategies
Altarum Institute

Altarum Institute is a non-profit research institute, focusing on improving health and health care. Altarum works with clients in many areas, and has recently written three reports for AHRQ on

- Interface design considerations

- Evaluation and use case framework

- Vendor practices and perspectives

(These reports are all available at http://healthit.ahrq.gov.)

Ms. Werner shared the common complaints her team heard in their study of health professionals' experiences with EHRs, as shown on this slide:

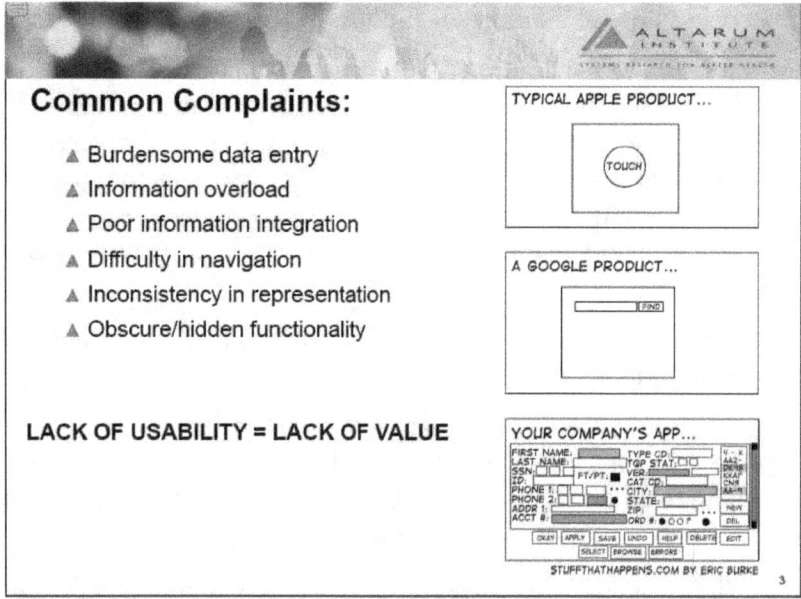

Vendors don't believe there are standards for health IT. They are borrowing standards from other domains, developing their own, trying to respond to users and to requirements such as CCHIT testing. All of this leads to vendors feeling pulled in many directions and confused.

Vendors are not communicating with each other. Formal usability testing is not being done, except for some large vendors. Vendors conduct focus groups and take in feedback from users, but vendors don't know much about – or understand – real usability testing. They think that usability = satisfaction.

Usability testing will increase as vendors see usability is seen as a competitive differentiator.

Vendors are willing to collaborate and share and use best practices.

So we need

- a framework
- objective measures
- communicate with vendors and the user community
- increase usability testing
- provide standards, guidelines, and best practices

Presenting the EHR within the provider and patient's digital lifestyle

Clifford Goldsmith, M.D.
Health Plan Industry Strategist,
Microsoft Corporation

Dr. Goldsmith added another message to the discussion: The world of health care is about to change. We are moving from health *information* technology to health *improvement* technology.

Reducing the cost of care will require changing from episodic care to continuous care and to involving patients more. We are moving to generations that use more technologies in different ways; we will have to work with the digital lifestyle of people who use short messaging systems, short attention spans.

Using his own weight-loss and health improvement experiences as an example, Goldsmith showed a wide array of web sites with different interfaces. He pointed out how difficult it would be for a physician to follow this patient's experience because the sites represent names, dates, charts, etc. differently.

He mentioned a Microsoft project to develop a common user interface with these tools:

- Guides for how to use systems
- Solution accelerators (tools for making it easier to build systems)
- Patient journey demonstrators (videos)

Usability, user experience, and clinician happiness: What's the connection?

Jacob Reider, M.D.
Chief Medical Informatics Officer
Allscripts

The people who buy systems in hospitals get input from computer people who don't have much connection to the actual users. We have to get them information from the actual users.

Dr. Reider showed a pyramid of six attributes of a system. From bottom to top, the attributes of this pyramid are:

- Functional
- Reliable

- Usable

- Convenient

- Pleasurable

- Meaningful

He pointed out that "Functional" is at the bottom. "Usable" is only part way up the pyramid. "Pleasurable" and "meaningful" are at the top. And he insisted that we have to get to pleasurable and meaningful.

The goal must be to give people a clear path and to help people stay on the right path in a system – to put up guard rails to help them – rather than to rely on alerts.

Usability perspectives from HIMSS

Edna Boone, M.A., C.P.H.I.M.S.
Senior Director, Health Information Systems
HIMSS

The mission of the Healthcare Information and Management Systems Society (HIMSS) is to lead health care transformation through effective use of health information technology. The organization has more than 30,000 individual members and more than 450 corporate members.

HIMSS now has a usability task force.

Ms. Boone reminded us that hospitals have to deal with not only federal requirements, but also with state and local requirements. In these tough economic times, hospitals will be taking advantage of the incentives to buy or upgrade now. We can't wait a long time for usability guidance because hospitals need it now.

HIMSS tracks EMR adoption with a seven-stage model. About 50 percent of hospitals are at stage 3 – moving into Computerized Physician Order Entry (CPOE) next.

Most hospitals have bought systems. The next few years will be mostly about customizing, configuring, implementing, and training. How do we get the people doing these post-purchase tasks to understand and engage in usability?

Usability is not only an issue for vendors – yes, vendors must build more usability in. But purchasers must also know how to gauge the usability of systems. End users must be engaged – must provide feedback. And the usability community must be constructive partners; they must understand that "perfection is the enemy of the good."

Boone described the activities of the HIMSS usability task force with this slide:

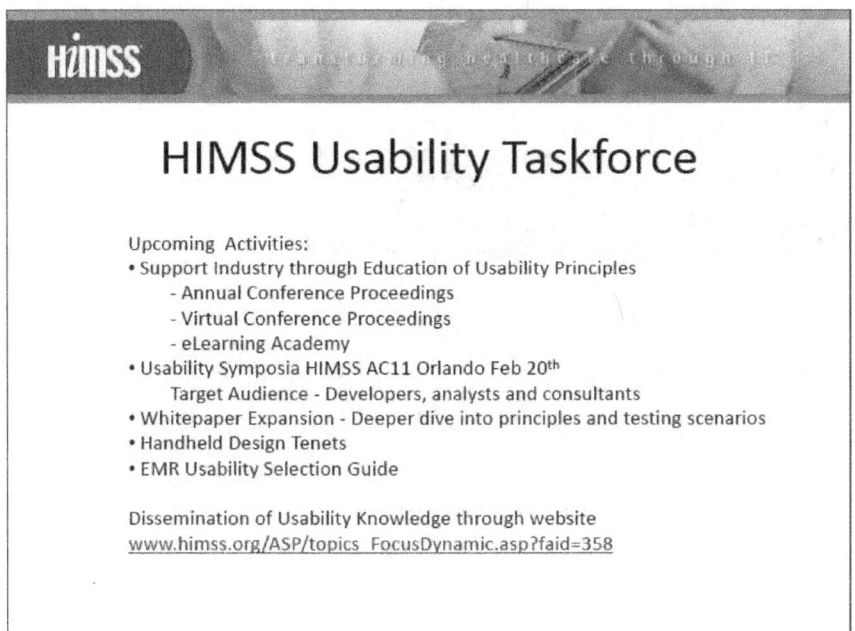

Building usability into purchasing and implementation processes

Rebecca Grayson
Healthcare IT Usability Consultant
Principal, User Reflections

Ms. Grayson is part of the HIMSS usability task force. Her talk focused on the work the task force has been doing to provide guidance on usability, particularly to the people in a medical practice who are purchasing or customizing health IT systems.

Long-term projects to develop best practices, guidelines, standards, and frameworks are very important. But they are on at least a two-year timeframe. And even after the projects are over, it will take longer for vendors to incorporate what the projects tell them.

Health care organizations must purchase and implement systems soon (to qualify for American Recovery and Reinvestment Act [ARRA] funds). But today usability evaluations are rarely performed; usability isn't in the equation for most health care organizations. We need actionable education now.

The HIMSS task force has just completed a guide, *Selecting an EMR for Your Practice: Evaluating Usability*. The guide, targeted to regional extension centers (RECs) and small medical practices, is marked as a draft because the task force sees it as just a first step. This slide shows what is in the guide:

Product Selection ...

- HIMSS usability evaluation guide contains:
  - "Usability" defined and explained
  - Usability principles clarified by EMR examples
  - Steps to include in the selection process
  - How to perform a simple hands-on usability test
  - Samples of:
    - Usability questions to include in an RFP
    - Usability testing scenarios
    - Post usability test questionnaires

The guide is a way for the people in a medical practice to judge the usability of a system they are considering (and not just to consider usability as subjective satisfaction). It is not meant as definitive, but as a way for practitioners to see how well a system is going to work in their practice.

Another important point that the HIMSS usability task force makes is that the usability of what is done in customization is also critical. They encourage applying usability guidelines, engaging usability professionals, and doing usability testing on any changes that are made to the system. They caution that extensive changes to a system may take away from the usability that was built in.

Q&A for the panel on Current State of EHRs and Need for Action

Dean Cross, Pittsburgh, PA, (audience)

Dr. Cross commented on some functionality he would like to see in an EHR: search that would allow him to see, for example, if lab data is ready or if new information has been introduced. He asked Dr. Patel if he had categorized and recorded the event when the EMR crashed. Patel responded that they record errors that affect patients and record problems that are caught downstream.

Matthew Quinn, AHRQ

Mr. Quinn posed this question to the panel: Dr. Koppel's presentation included a slide about how vendors could be putting up barriers preventing new vendors if regulations for usability and meaningful use set very high expectations. Quinn asked whether we are already too late for the coming wave of ARRA-HITECH stimulus-funded EHR adoption and "the cake is already baked without the flour in it and raising regulations would essentially be like trying to pound flour into a cake that is already baked."

Koppel responded that hospitals that have spent significant amounts of money on an existing EHR system are typically unwilling to ask their boards for more money to buy a new system, even if their current system is proving to be challenging.

Dr. Goldsmith, however, answered that companies could offer components for specific aspects of a system – such as a uniform date and time widget, how the name and age are displayed, etc. In this way, we could introduce usability in small steps.

Panel 2: Measuring and Reporting Usability

In the second session of short talks, we again heard from six speakers.

Methods of measuring usability

Charles Friedman, Ph.D.
Chief Scientific Officer
Office of the National Coordinator for Health Information Technology

Dr. Friedman reminded us that there are a range of methods for evaluating systems, including both qualitative and quantitative measures. He urged us not to close the door too quickly on any method.

Qualitative measures have value in the richness of the data – "thick description." And rigorous qualitative measures exist. It may be "soft" data, but it is also highly meaningful. With qualitative measures, you often ask a variety of experts to review a system (the "art criticism" model). For EHRs, you would want experts with both health care and IT backgrounds.

You should not expect experts to completely agree, but you get very useful and informative insights.

Quantitative measures give you "hard" data, but that data may be less meaningful because it may be less obvious what causes problems and how to fix the problems. With quantitative measures, you must

- Agree on what to measure and what result is "better"
- Create controlled conditions for measurement
- Identify a proper range of cases
- Control for other factors
- Recruit appropriate users at different levels of experience
- Collect comparable data across systems.

Health IT design and usability: Myths and realities

Ben-Tzion Karsh, Ph.D.
Associate Professor, Industrial and System Engineering
University of Wisconsin

Dr. Karsh presented and refuted nine myths about usability:

1. Myth: Usability is only affected by software design.

    No. Many other elements affect usability, including: workflow, time pressures, physical space layout, lighting, policies of use, and more. That means that a system can work well in a lab setting, and, thus, be certified, but still not be usable in practice.

2. Myth: Making software screens and layouts simple and consistent leads to usability.

    No. Those are necessary, but not sufficient, conditions. Content matters.

3. Myth: Dense data displays lead to cognitive overload. We need very simple displays.

    No. Experts are used to dense displays.

4. Myth: Health IT should integrate into clinical workflow.

    But what does that mean if workflow is emergent? We don't necessarily want to just put current (often, poor) workflows into new systems. We need flexible systems that support different workflows and quick retrieval of data.

5. Myth: User-centered design means giving users what they want.

    No. User-centered design means involving users, listening to them, but also applying skills and knowledge of expert usability specialists and designers. What users say they want may not be the best way to help them achieve their goals.

    We need an ongoing, continuous research program. Other complex systems that humans use – for example, aviation – has a continuous program of human factors research.

6. Myth: Usability is the goal.

    No. The goal is to design systems that support clinicians' ability to provide high quality and safe care. Usability is an attribute of a system that contributes to the true goal.

7. Myth: Usability measurement is subjective.

    We have hard metrics for usability. But people's perception of usability is important, too. "Perception is what drives action."

8. Myth: There are no usability standards for health IT.

    We have design standards in human factors on many issues that are relevant to health IT systems.

9. Myth: Usability means EHRs that are so intuitive you don't need training.

    No. We have to recognize that these are complex systems and require training. A complex system does not have to be complicated. But if we continue to not have time for training, we are in trouble.

Karsh recommended that ONC create an advisory board to focus on usability issues, as we see on this slide:

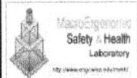

Implications

- The ONC should consider establishing a federal *clinician cognitive work* (or usability) advisory board that can help them to think about meaningful use, EHRs, CDS, etc from the viewpoint of supporting clinician cognitive work

Evidence-based usability practice

Kai Zheng, Ph.D.
Assistant Professor, Information Systems and Health Informatics
University of Michigan

Dr. Zheng reiterated earlier speakers' point that many usability issues do not emerge in laboratory testing. He also pointed out that usability "issues" may be temporary, as users simply do not want to give up old ways of working. The system may be perceived as unusable because it is trying to change people's ways of working.

He raised the idea of using patterns based on Christopher Alexander's book on Pattern Languages (Alexander, Ishikawa, and Silverstein, 1977). Patterns and pattern libraries have become very popular among software designers. A pattern is a known solution to a recurring situation, so that, instead of inventing a new way of doing something each time the situation arises, the designer selects the appropriate pattern from the system's pattern library. This promotes consistency; and, if the patterns have been tested, it promotes usability in the system.

Zheng also added to the workshop's list of resources, mentioning:

- Tidwell, *Designing Interfaces*, O'Reilly
- www.usability.gov
- Research-Based Web Design and Usability Guidelines
- Air Force Guidelines
- Apple's Human Interface Guidelines
- Microsoft's Health Common User Interface guidelines

Zheng concluded by suggesting that we can have evidence-based usability practice by gathering what is known already about good interface design and by having an ongoing program of formative evaluation that continues to find evidence-based practice as new technologies emerge.

Methods of measuring usability

Scott Lind
Director of User Experience
Soarian, Siemens Healthcare

Mr. Lind raised the issue of whether it is wise to measure usability with a single score. He questions whether that gives a true picture of the usability of a system.

He described a series of studies in which different teams got quite different results for the same usability test. What happens in a usability test depends on many factors, including the tasks, the participants, and the context. We would have to work very hard to get good representative tasks that really tested the usability of the system as a whole. What is usable for a nurse could be very different than what is usable for a physician. We need to take a broader view of usability than a single score allows us to do.

Lind also pointed out that usability and safety are two separate attributes that overlap. He suggests starting with tasks and participants in that overlap, as being most important for systems.

Impacting usability with appropriate user-based research

Janey Barnes, Ph.D.
Human Factors Specialist
User-View, Inc.

Dr. Barnes returned us to the theme that Edna Boone and Rebecca Grayson expounded in the first panel session: the need for usability education now. Vendors and health information specialists who equate usability with user satisfaction need to learn what usability really is.

She also reminded us again that usability is not just cognitive. It's about the physical, social, organizational components; and that to test usability of a system, we must take a systems-level approach.

For appropriate usability measures, Barnes also explained that we must match usability techniques and measures to the research questions, as shown in this slide:

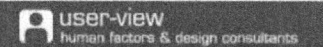

Appropriate Usability Methods

- Applied Behavioral Science
    - with physical, cognitive and social and organizational components (even HIT includes all these components)
    - Systems require a systems level approach
- Match the Research Method → the Research Question → How the Data will be Used
    - Formative / Summative
    - Informal / Formal
    - Data for Selection

July 2010   4

Reviewing different methods, she suggested that we are not going to get by with discount usability methods in health IT. We are going to have to use formal human factors methods.

Barnes' third point was that we must find ways to share findings from usability – and sharing in ways that are appropriate for each audience.

CCHIT's one-score rating was a good start. The organization was amazing to move so fast. But with 90 percent of those who show their ratings receiving five stars (out of five), we need to move beyond the initial CCHIT method.

Usability testing at CCHIT

Alisa Ray, M.S.
Executive Director
CCHIT

The Certification Commission for Health Information Technology (CCHIT) is an independent 501c(3) organization that helps to accelerate the adoption of health IT. CCHIT has been testing EHRs for about six years; but until recently, usability was not part of their test method.

Feeling that they needed to get started in usability, they found a way to put measures of usability into their existing testing method for ambulatory care systems. That testing method is to have a vendor walk a panel of three jurors through scenarios (preset by CCHIT) with the vendor's software. All sessions are conducted remotely with each juror watching and listening from their own venue. The jurors, who are clinicians and informatics specialists with lots of experience of many EHR systems, assess the system step-by-step, voting at each step.

The jurors have score sheets that they use to evaluate the systems on a number of criteria. Within the time constraints of this process, CCHIT was able to add usability questions to the scoring sheets, as explained on this slide:

Rating Model

- Jurors are given a series of questionnaires to create the rating of usability based on observations.

  - After Scenario Questionnaire (ASQ) – jurors rate perceived efficiency (time and effort), learnability, and confidence after viewing scenarios

    - 4 questions after each scenario – 16 overall

  - Perceived Usability Questionnaire (PERUSE)– jurors rate screen-level design attributes based on reasonably observable characteristics

    - 20 questions divided among each of the scenarios; Jurors are allowed to revisit answers to these questions

  - System Usability Survey (SUS) – jurors rate the assessment of usability, and satisfaction with the application

    - 10 questions after all four scenarios have been demonstrated

 CCHIT
© 2009   Slide 7   October 2, 2009

Ms. Ray sees what CCHIT is doing as a first step in putting usability into the certification inspection. For now, the usability rating does not affect the certification outcome. However, vendors get a rating (1 – 5 stars) for usability, and they get feedback on each item in the scoring. Of the 26 vendors who have been through the process with the usability component: 2 achieved 3 stars, 7 achieved 4 stars, and 17 achieved 5 stars.

Q&A for the panel on Measuring and Reporting Usability

Dean Cross, Pittsburgh, PA, (audience)

For Ms. Ray: Where is the CCHIT lab located?

Alisa Ray, CCHIT

The testing is done virtually where the jurors can see the vendor's product screen as the vendor goes through each scenario. Virtual testing like this is cost effective, takes less setup, reduces travel time, and is very efficient. In the new government rules, the government has said that virtual inspection is the preferred method.

Ross Koppel, University of Pennsylvania

For Dr. Karsh: Related to the need for training, a difference between pilots and doctors is that for pilots the training is on their primary tasks. For doctors, using the EMR is not their primary job. Also, doctors may practice in three or four different hospitals; they don't want to have to be trained on that many different systems.

Ben-Tzion Karsh, University of Wisconsin

Dr. Karsh said he understands and appreciates the problem Dr. Koppel raised, but reiterated that we have to get out of the mindset that we are going to have systems people can walk up to and intelligently start using without training.

Panel 3: "Points of Pain" – Addressing EHR User Disparities

In the third panel, we heard from five speakers.

Accessibility and health IT

David Baquis
Accessibility Specialist
U.S. Access Board

Mr. Baquis spoke without slides. He reminded us that accessibility means removing barriers that make it difficult or impossible for people with disabilities to use a product such as EHRs.

Accessibility complements usability; but accessibility is different from usability. Accessibility is rooted in the civil rights movement and is a civil rights issue.

What problems might people with disabilities have related to health IT? They might have problems

- Using the software to enter information

- Navigating a web site to get to a health record

- Using a PDF

- Taking an e-learning course

Section 508 makes us think about many modalities: videos, telecommunication products, handhelds, information kiosks as you might find in a pharmacy. We are not only talking about patients with disabilities, but also about clinicians, who might be disabled from the beginning of their careers or become disabled; about other people in the stakeholder chain, such as people in the insurance industry.

Recommendations:

- Elevate accessibility to be a top concern, at the same level as security, interoperability, and usability

- Include accessibility in all activities: strategic plan, standards, certification, etc.

Creating an inclusive infrastructure to allow affordable access across technologies, disabilities, and ages

Gregg Vanderheiden, Ph.D.
Professor and Director, Trace Center
University of Wisconsin

Dr. Vanderheiden reminded us that communication is a critical aspect of health records. The people who must use these records include people with the attributes on this slide:

Who are these users?

- People with **disabilities**
    (visual, hearing, physical, cognitive)
- People who are **older**
- People who use **different language** from the equipment
- People who are **not technically inclined**
- People with **literacy** problems
- People who are **sick**
- People who are **tired**
- People who are **panicked**

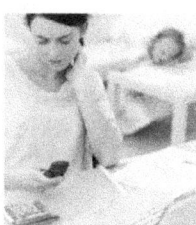

But developers are very technically inclined and develop on the assumption that users are just like them. We need simple and obvious interfaces that work for people who may be in the situations listed on this slide:

What do they We need?

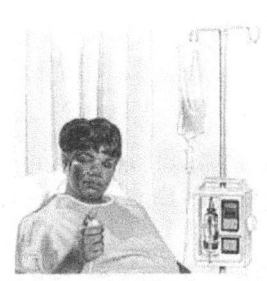

- Simple – to the point of Obvious
- Usable with poor vision
- Usable with arthritis
- Usable without vision
- Usable in a noisy environment
- Error resistant when you are tired
    panicked, or rushed

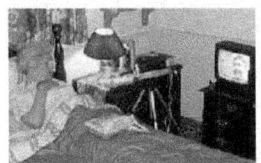 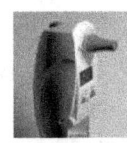

Vanderheiden explained that we need to

- find ways to help people conform to the guidelines more easily

- have standard formats so underlying data is the same even if system differs

- allow individuals to have the interface that works for them and have that interface apply across systems

- incorporate email, chat, and pictures with our health IT systems

- make interfaces that give people what they need

He described an ongoing project to create a National Public Inclusive Infrastructure (NPII). This is a coalition of academic / government / industry, working with international standards that will allow any system to be transformed into an interface that is individually prescribed. The individual's profile is securely stored without personal identifying information and tells products how to change to fit that individual's needs. This would allow companies to create products that can adapt to all without having to design a product for all these different groups.

The SHARP-C approach to EHR usability

Jaijie Zhang, Ph.D.
Dr. Doris L. Ross Professor & Associated Dean of Research
University of Texas Health Science Center at Houston

ONC identified six challenges to adoption and meaningful use of health IT, based on an earlier report by the National Research Council. ONC has funded six projects to deal with these challenges. Dr. Zhang is the Principal Investigator of one of these projects, a nine-institution consortium on a four-year mission to develop a unified framework for EHR usability.

The framework they have developed is called UFuRT: User, Function, Representation, Task Analysis. It provides an overview of what you need to do either to evaluate or develop a system:

- Understand the users (develop personas)

- Get a detailed understanding of the work the system must allow the users to accomplish (functions, work ontology) and the constraints the system must account for – this is independent of any implementation / interface

- Prototype an implementation

- Do task analysis of what people do and what the system does (evaluate the prototype for the users and the work)

They have used the framework to evaluate EHR systems and to compare systems. And UFuRT can be used to design new systems.

Zhang's final slide shows that usability must be considered a combination of how useful it is (the work a system allows people to accomplish) and how usable it is (the interactions and interface it implements for people to do their tasks).

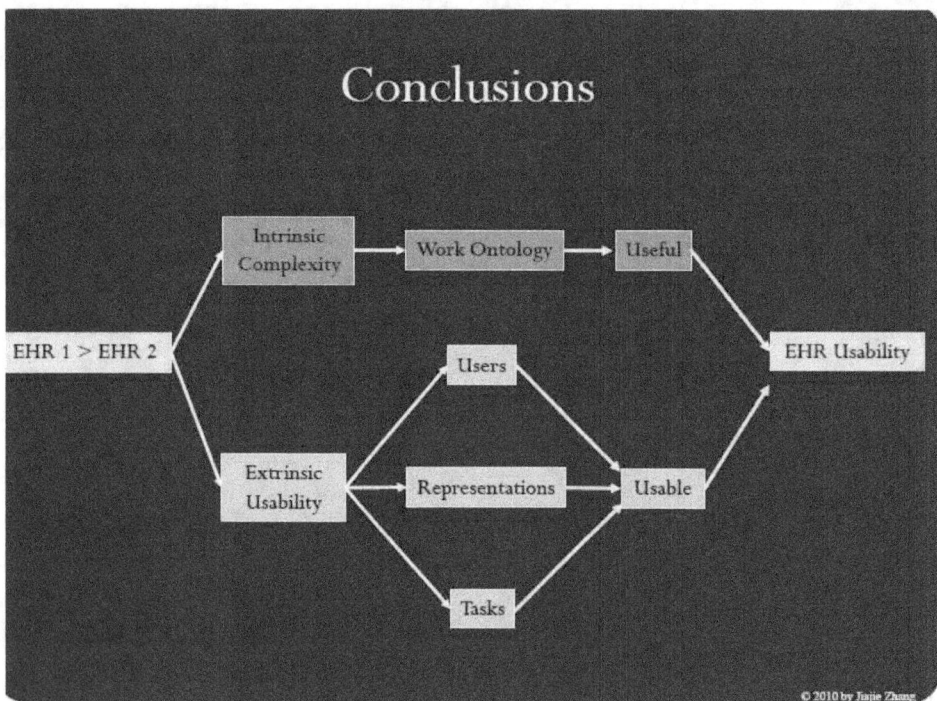

TeachEHR: Who's training the clinical workforce

Juan Gilbert, Ph.D.
Professor and Chair of Human Centered Computing
Clemson University

Dr. Gilbert addressed the issue of training, but from a different perspective than earlier speakers. His concern is how to train *future* clinical practitioners, such as students in Clemson University's School of Nursing. He raised the three questions on this slide:

$$\left[\right]$$

TeachEHR

- As EHR/PHR systems are deployed, who's training clinical practitioners?

- What competencies should future practitioners be taught?

- What system or platform should be used?

As Gilbert explained, teaching any one existing system would be problematic: Which one would you choose? How would you pay for a commercial system? How would you work with a system that was not developed for the purpose of training people?

So Gilbert and his colleagues at Clemson University developed their own system specifically for teaching a set of competencies that they determined were most important. It is not a complete EHR. Examples of competencies they are using the system to teach include:

- Identify and maintain a patient record

- Manage medication administration

- Manage a patient's history

They also want the system focus on training – that is, to have functions such as the ability to track students' performance.

Gilbert also expressed concern about problems in helping people transfer their skills and knowledge from one system to another. He cited automobiles and programming languages as two examples of domains in which it is fairly easy to transfer knowledge from one system to another. He also cited voting as a domain in which we have seen very real problems due to poor usability because the technology got ahead of usability, as we see on this slide:

Usable Health Records

- EHR should be usable and accessible

- Lack of usability and accessibility will result in
  - Lack of trust
  - Potential abuse

- Lessons from electronic voting
  - No election has been proven to have been hacked; however, usability has altered the outcome of an election

Usability is more than user satisfaction: 10 principles of EMR usability

Jeffrey Belden, M.D.
Associate Professor of Clinical Family & Community Medicine
University of Missouri

Dr. Belden introduced himself as an "evangelist of EHR usability." He urged us to "say it with pictures." In his talk, Belden showed how images can be used to illustrate principles of EHR usability. He also urged us to develop visual style guides and to conduct research on the visual display of usability.

Belden described and visually depicted these 10 principles:

- Simplicity: Depending on the task at hand, a doctor may want different views of the data.

- Naturalness: How well does the task correspond to our mental model. His example allows doctors to indicate a body part on an image of a person rather than dig down through layers of word-based menus.

- Consistency: An image can show how to place parts of a screen.

- Minimize cognitive load: Display the level of information that the specific user needs for the specific task.

- Efficient interactions: His visual example is a dashboard for clinicians that brings together what they need for a specific task.

- Forgiveness: Good error messages. (His example is a very visual example of what not to do.)

- Feedback: He shows three visual ways – good, better, even better – of how to display feedback.

- Effective use of language: He shows an example of adjusting the language identifying medicines with different displays for doctors and patients.

- Effective information presentation: He shows a visual display of sorting and highlighting information from a list where different specialists would be most interested in different items in the list.

- Preservation of context: He uses the dashboard again as an example.

Looking at how visual some style guides are for interface development, Belden cited:

- Research-Based Web Design and Usability Guidelines from www.usability.gov with the visual scales for importance and strength of evidence; each guideline is accompanied by an example.

- Microsoft's Common User Interface guidelines which often show how to do something and how not to do it.

- UI Design Patterns as an example of one of many web sites that show design patterns for user interfaces.

- Apple's User Interface Guidelines, which also shows examples.

We need further research on how well different visual techniques work.

Panel 4: Defining Federal Strategy: ONC, NIST, AHRQ, and FDA Usability Collective Efforts

Svetlana Lowry from NIST, Matthew Quinn from AHRQ, and Ron Kaye from the Food and Drug Administration (FDA) spoke in this session.

Building a technical framework for usability and accessibility of EHRs

Svetlana Lowry, Ph.D.
Human Factors Lead, Health IT
NIST

In speaking about NIST's plans and strategies for this very important program, Dr. Lowry said that NIST's task is to establish technical standards for usability and accessibility of electronic health records.

She pointed out that two critical aspects of EHRs are that they must

- Promote the ability of clinicians to perform routine tasks

- Ensure that the user interface does not lead to critical errors

Lowry suggested that while user satisfaction is important, satisfaction doesn't stop errors from occurring. She urged attendees to help assure that systems that are certified

- Help clinicians deliver the right treatment to the right patient at the right time

- Be accessible to all who use them

- Account for other factors that can lead to subpar performance, such as English as a second language, low literacy, and stress

We must be primarily concerned with how EHRs do with respect to

- Data handling

- Error handling

- Utility and usability

Data handling: Lowry pointed out that, with EHRs, we are really talking about a meta-system where data exchange and data retrieval are critical across systems. Therefore, we must have data presented in consistent and intuitive formats.

Error handling: Lowry mentioned that for certification, we must know how many errors users make, how severe the errors are, and how easily users recover from errors.

Utility and usability: As other speakers had also done, Lowry insisted that we must consider both of these together. A system that does not allow users to do the tasks they need to do has no utility – and, therefore, is not usable. A system that has the functionality but that leads to lack of task success or high error rates has no usability – and therefore, cannot / will not be used.

Lowry pointed out that we must find out at what point the complexity of a task causes the user to fail to complete the task as intended or worse to fail to complete the task and not to be aware of it. We must find out what causes users to lose faith in the reliability of the system or lose confidence in the system. We must learn what causes users to perform incorrectly or to perform unnecessary actions.

Although we know a lot about human factors, we must still research specifics in the context of EHRs. Lowry said that NIST will conduct extensive human factors research to establish standards for certification and pass / fail criteria for testing to those standards. The end goal is to have standards and a protocol for pass / fail testing that can be shown to be reliable and valid so the protocol can be performed consistently across multiple laboratories.

Lowry also added her personal opinion that the test methods must include actual user performance measuring accuracy, success in task completion, and freedom from critical errors. She pointed out that while timing may be important for efficiency, it may not be as critical for pass / fail criteria as task success; and with laboratory-based testing, measures of time may have less relevance for real-world performance than measures of accuracy and task success.

AHRQ research efforts to assess and improve the usability of EHRs

Matthew Quinn, M.B.A.
Special Expert, Health IT
AHRQ

AHRQ's mission is to improve the quality, safety, efficiency, and effectiveness of health care for all Americans.

AHRQ is a small agency: 300 people. AHRQ focuses on long-term and system-wide improvements of health care quality and effectiveness. AHRQ looks at systems; not at specific diseases or specific populations.

Quinn discussed one project that AHRQ has been involved in that focused on the best ways to visually display data. Research like that is important because people adopt systems that they like to use, that are not painful to use, that give them value without overloading them.

AHRQ is also concerned with the safe and effective use of systems, with not having system-introduced errors.

And AHRQ is concerned with innovation. Quinn suggested that standards do not stifle innovation; just the opposite. In fact, lots of innovation is happening, but it's not getting into commercial systems. So one issue is how we get these innovations into commercial systems.

Quinn asked: How do we shift the paradigm from systems that are just documenting things to systems that help clinicians make better, faster decisions.

While there seem to be large gaps in knowledge and practice, perhaps there isn't from what we are hearing today; but then the question is what is relevant from other disciplines to apply to health IT and what is not relevant.

Giving credit to James Bell Associates and the Altarum Institute, Quinn mentioned three reports (all available at www.healthit.ahrq.gov):

- *EHR Usability: Evaluation and Use Case Framework*

- *EHR Usability: Interface Design Considerations*

- *EHR Usability: Vendor Practices and Perspectives*

AHRQ put together an expert panel to consider what is known elsewhere that would be relevant for Health IT. That resulted in recommendations for policies and research. AHRQ is also funding a project to synthesize available guidelines into an objective toolkit that clinicians can use to evaluate the usability of health IT for primary care.

Enhancing user performance and avoiding safety problems through analysis, discovery, prioritization, and design

Ron Kaye, M.A.
Human Factors and Device Use Safety Team Leader
FDA

Mr. Kaye explained that his work is primarily looking at human factors of submissions of medical devices that are seeking FDA approval. He usually is looking at hardware devices, but sometimes the devices are entirely software.

As a human factors (HF) specialist, Kaye knows that usability is best when it is built into the device rather than added on as Quinn said earlier, like "pounding flour into the cake after it has been baked."

In Kaye's job, the primary considerations are safe and effective use. To judge that, you must consider environments, users, and the device itself, as Kaye showed in this slide of the model that his division uses:

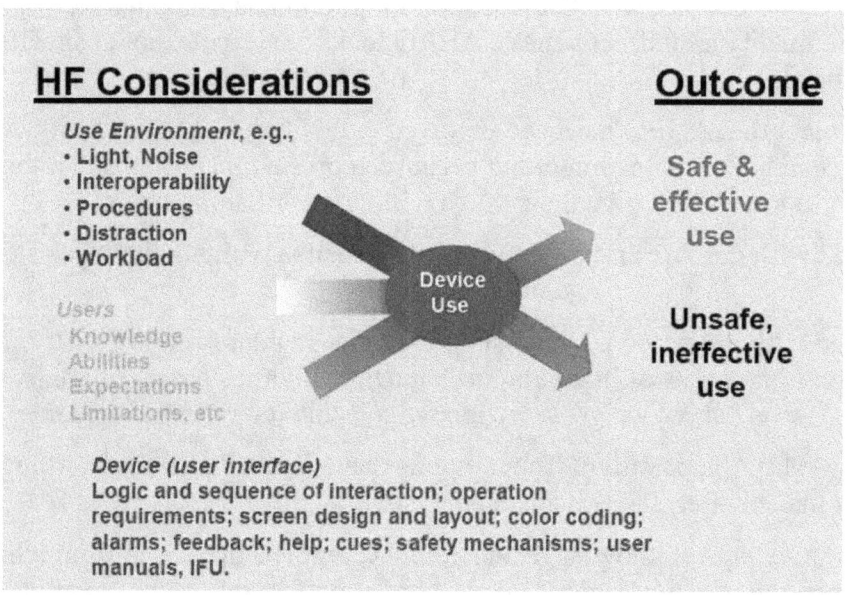

Kaye also explained that it is very important to know about the errors users make. However, it is often difficult to get that information with current reporting systems. Users sometimes don't even know what they did or what happened to cause the error. And they don't know how to communicate the problem. That makes it difficult for human factors experts like Kaye to give good feedback to the device manufacturers. So a need is to refine ways of getting that information.

He then described a human factors / usability approach for manufacturers to follow, which begins by taking into account the factors on the slide shown above. The approach includes urging manufacturers to involve users early and throughout the design process, to evaluate the device with actual users doing actual tasks iteratively throughout design.

Kaye pointed out that with any device you are testing for both anticipated difficulties and the unanticipated difficulties that will inevitably show up. Identifying those unanticipated difficulties are part of the real value of usability testing. While he stressed the importance of gathering subjective data from users, Kaye also stressed that user preference does not necessarily equal optimal design.

He also urged manufacturers to test tasks of low frequency and to consider atypical users and use, which are often overlooked in human factors / usability evaluations.

Kaye concluded by giving us a list of international human factors standards, as shown on this slide:

National and International HF Standards applicable to HF Medical Devices

- ANSI/AAMI/ISO 14971:2001 Risk Management
- ANSI/AAMI HE74: 2001, Human factors design process for medical devices
- ANSI/AAMI HE75: 2010, Human factors design principles for medical devices (in progress)
- IEC 62366 Usability
- IEC 60601-1-6 Usability
- IEC 60601-1-8, Alarm Systems

4. Open Discussion:
Recommendations and Next Steps

For the last two hours of the day, everyone in the room was invited to participate in an open discussion that focused on these four questions:

- What should be the role of the federal government / industry / academia in improving the usability and accessibility of EHRs?

- How can the federal government work to improve the availability of objective information about the usability and accessibility of EHRs?

- Based on the day's presentations, what are the key breakthroughs necessary to advance the usability and accessibility of EHRs? How can the federal government facilitate these breakthroughs?

- What are the key needs of private sector efforts to improve usability and accessibility of EHRs that the government can support?

The moderator began by posing the first of these questions to start the discussion.

In this chapter, panel members are named with their affiliations. Audience members who spoke were asked to identify themselves and their affiliations. Where the audiotape is clear enough to find the person on the list of attendees, we have included the person's name and affiliation as well as an indication that this was someone from the audience. Otherwise, we have identified the comment simply as "audience."

Edna Boone, HIMMS

Industry is looking to government for

- Leadership like this meeting

- Continued research

- Standards

- Certification

- Resources such as those proposed by AHRQ and NIST

She is concerned about timelines, asking what is really doable in the near future (next two years). And then how do we build towards standards and certification in the longer term.

For immediate needs, she suggests we must educate vendors and clinicians and equip implementers with usability and accessibility principles.

Greg Vanderheiden, Trace Center, University of Wisconsin

The key part needs to be leadership in standards and interoperability. We need to separate the interface level from the layers underneath. If we had a standard platform that allows for innovation and competition on the interface level, you don't have to replace entire system. He would look to the government for leadership on these underlying standards – standard formats, data standards.

Charles Friedman, ONC

ONC has funded four SHARP projects. We heard about one of them in the short presentations. Another is the SMART project at Boston Children's Hospital. (SMART = Substitutable Medical Applications, Reusable Technologies). It is researching just what Dr. Vanderheiden is looking for.

The idea is to develop a platform architecture that will take plug-ins of substitutable applications and that could be customized for specific users and could follow them around from place to place. The project was funded in April 2010; the platform is expected to be available in 2012.

Greg Vanderheiden, Trace Center, University of Wisconsin

Urged quick results and a user interface architecture, too.

Ross Koppel, University of Pennsylvania

The greatest need is for interoperability. Without interoperability, an EHR is like a standalone fax machine with no other fax machines to send information to.

Dr. Koppel also urged the government to get information about usability out there. As he said, "We know stuff about usability." We don't have to do a lot of research to know what's wrong with many of these systems.

Rebecca Grayson, User Reflections

Great concern is the timeframe. Purchasing and implementation is happening now. We need to educate vendors and buyers and implementers now.

Ms. Grayson would look to the government for leadership and collaboration in education now. She urged increased government staffing for health IT resources that would give health care organizations education on usability and accessibility now.

Robyne Kenton, Vision Foundry, audience

Ms. Kenton identified herself as a user experience (UX) specialist. She suggested that the government create a portal, a UX framework that EHR vendors could plug into. She urged the government to standardize primary keys and context, to set conventions (for example, if people expect to see search functionality in the upper left, then leave it in the upper left). This would still allow users to customize and allow vendors to compete with upgrades.

Matthew Quinn, AHRQ

Agreed that separating the user interface from the rest of the EHR system components is good idea. But he does not think vendors would use the portal unless they were forced to. And he wonders why no one had gone after this market opportunity if it really does exist.

Ben-Tzion Karsh, University of Wisconsin

We should not use usability rankings; we should not be giving stars. The vendors know what they will be tested for, so they can make sure they are okay for the test. That does not indicate real usability.

Rather, we should have transparent usability assessment with real data from real users. For example, buyers should be able to look up in a table and find how fast users are able to find what they need (for example, lab data) in different systems. We should have objective data for real comparisons – both time data and satisfaction numbers.

To do that, we have to determine what we are designing for and set usability standards, for example, that a clinician will be able to get to a patient's lab results within x seconds.

Scott Lind, Siemens Healthcare

Vendors have competing calls on their resources. For each release cycle, they have to decide where to invest their resources. We all have to understand that this is a challenge for vendors – deciding how to prioritize, deciding what to invest in.

Jiajie Zhang, University of Texas

Dr. Zhang raised the issue of international coordination. He asked whether there is any activity with organizations in other countries to get together and do something together so as not to duplicate work.

Charles Friedman, ONC

Dr. Friedman indicated that one of his responsibilities at ONC is to oversee a small global e-health component. Health IT is not a U.S. phenomenon. It's a global revolution and many countries are far ahead of the U.S. Some countries have 100 percent EHR use in primary care. We have a lot to learn from them, and we should pursue that learning both government to government and through other associations and non-government entities.

When asked which countries have very high use of electronic records in primary care, Friedman named England, Sweden, Denmark, Holland, and Australia.

David Baquis, U.S. Access Board

Mr. Baquis noted that they had four international members on a recent advisory board for communication technology standards, representing Japan, Australia, Canada, and the European Commission. International harmonization is high on the Access Board's agenda. They hope that when other countries create standards, they will share them with the U.S., and they recognize that vendors don't want to have to create different products to different standards for different countries. Baquis sees health information technology as a subset of communication technology standards.

Charles Webster, Encounter Pro, (audience)

Mr. Webster pointed out the connection between workflow management and usability. He would like to see the government include and encourage more of this workflow management technology migrate into the health care sector. There is a conversion going on in business process management from a traditional business-centric workflow to a more human-centered workflow. Not "doing by design'" – forcing people to follow the way the product is designed, but "design by doing" – where the workflow emerges from the work as people do it.

Juan Gilbert, Clemson University

Dr. Gilbert points out that not all current workflow practices in health care are optimal. We must be cautious about making systems that perpetuate poor workflow practices. Webster argues for plasticity in the software to allow for starting with something that will not produce culture shock but that can be smoothed into better workflow practices.

Clifford Goldsmith, Microsoft

The move toward patient-centered medical home care is starting to drive work flow. We need tools in these systems for having medical care plans for individuals, which is, in fact, all about workflow. For example, need customer relationship management tools inside of EHRs, EMRs.

Dean Cross, Practitioner, Pittsburg (audience)

Dr. Cross suggests that we now have a meaningful use law on devices with limited usability. He suggests that the U.S. government is spending money on devices that are not usable and wants to see a moratorium on government spending for deploying devices until usability catches up.

Jon White, AHRQ

While there are issues with EHRs, they represent progress. With EHRs, we are catching 50 percent more errors in order entries than we do with paper. While the tools are not perfect, we can still use them as we progress even further. We don't want to stop progress. All systems have benefits and risks.

Ross Koppel, University of Pennsylvania

Dr. Koppel does not want his research to be interpreted as anti-health IT. While he may point out places where, for example, alerts are largely ignored, EHRs have the advantage of being able to move information in multiple directions fast, to catch errors in other ways. The advantages of the systems are extraordinary.

Jacob Reider, Allscripts

Dr. Reider talked about how technology has evolved over time. But the advance in other industries, such as the auto industry, has been slow. So the question is how do we accelerate this process for health IT? How can the government be an accelerant? He suggested that perhaps the government's role should be to provide a framework, an infrastructure, that is like "chicken wire" where the vendors can put their own paper mâché over the chicken wire.

He also believes that EHRs are good; they have improved health care; they do improve health care. He would not practice without one.

Neil Patel, Special Care Center

Dr. Patel reiterated the need for safety, for interoperability, for an accelerant, for a framework. He thinks that the framework, the infrastructure, the chicken wire is already in existence. He suggests that the government should require that for ARRA funding, vendors must pull back the paper mâché to reveal what the infrastructure they are using looks like. Perhaps the database should be open and not proprietary. He argued that we don't have time to build a new infrastructure, new platforms. Hundreds of platforms exist. If we opened the platforms, new companies would come in and innovate for better safety, better interoperability, and better usability.

Rebecca Grayson, User Reflections

Picking up on the theme of chicken wire on which more is laid over time: Can we have preliminary usability guidelines without waiting two years? Can we have quick tools while the AHRQ toolkit is being developed?

Bettijoyce Lide, NIST

Ms. Lide thanked Ms. Grayson for her comments. She said that NIST is a public - private partnership, which is why NIST is proud to be one of the sponsors of this workshop. NIST wants comments before, during, and after research. Everything NIST does through contracts, grants, in-house will be open for public comment in a variety of venues. Today is just the beginning of a dialogue. She urged people to email NIST, visit NIST, etc. The federal government does not do or want to do work that the private sector can and wants to do alone. The government works on infrastructure and in collaboration.

Svetlana Lowry, NIST

Dr. Lowry said that she hears and agrees with discussants that something needs to happen now to improve usability and accessibility. What the government can do is provide guidance to industry on what is important for user-centered design and usability. NIST has launched two grants that will help with this work. Deliverables will be coming shortly. Within one to two months, NIST will have a guide on human factors to prevent health IT disparities and a guide on human factors principles to help vendors with design.

David Baquis, U.S. Access Board

As answer to the question of what the role of the federal government should be in health IT, Mr. Baquis says: Serve as the model of governance of accessibility.

Let's help vendors get it right first. We have the Section 508 standards. Vendors could have been using them for the last decade. What we need to do now is spread the word that those are standards.

Also, we need to think "accessibility." Disabled people are not satisfied that the market is driving accessibility. That's why we have laws requiring accessibility. This is the 20th anniversary of the Americans for Disabilities Act. We should be pulling together recommendations from other workshops with those from this workshop and have a central repository for these recommendations.

John Smelcer, Fairfield Professionals, (audience)

Mr. Smelcer identified himself as a user experience professional. He said that user experience professionals know how to design usable systems. But when an IT clinician is making a decision about an EMR, functionality almost always trumps usability.

This seems like a fundamental problem. While you can use market forces to improve the value and importance of usability in EMRs, experience in other industries shows that you need government oversight and requirements. He cited the automobile industry as an example where safety was achieved by the government requiring seat belts, air bags, crash standards, etc, He suggested that the government needs to similarly impose usability and safety standards on the health IT community.

Jiajie Zhang, University of Texas

Dr. Zhang commented that in their SHARP project that are melding functionality and usability so people will not have to choose between them.

Juan Gilbert, Clemson University

Dr. Gilbert suggested that the pain of working with 'unusable' EHR systems needs to be highlighted. The pain needs to be felt. He wants to see usability made more prominent in legislators' minds and asks about advocacy groups.

Ginny Redish, Redish & Associates (the moderator)

Dr. Redish mentioned that there are professional societies of usability specialists: the Human Factors and Ergonomics Society and the Usability Professionals' Association.

Janine Purcell, IT Safety Office, U.S. Department of Veterans Affairs, (audience)

The U.S. Department of Veterans Affairs (VA) has an extensive set of components for an EHR, perhaps the most comprehensive aggregation of EHRs in the country. Her office gets issues that are encountered in using these EHRs in VA hospitals. Issues are flagged for actual or potential impact on patient safety.

They have a process for taking issues, assigning a risk score to them, prioritizing them for fixing, trying to fix them, and conducting post-market surveillance. So, the VA has a structure in place for change with policies and procedures in place. If issues can't be fixed, the VA notifies the public and end users to help prevent errors or danger.

She suggests that rather than throw out the technology, you have a process like this for continuous improvement.

Matthew Quinn, AHRQ

Mr. Quinn noted that every vendor has a way of capturing incidents and upgrade requests, but perhaps the process could be more formal. We could have a common format, a common taxonomy. Perhaps we could start with the VA's system.

Quinn and Ms. Purcell agreed that it's sometimes hard to get the whole story of what happened. Her office follows up with medical providers but it's still often hard after the fact to get the whole story. They have tried to create a template of good questions for people to report issues.

Kai Zhang, University of Michigan

Need to get vendors to move from reporting of usability issues to pay attention to these issues and build to avoid them. He suggests social media as a way to get and share information.

Audience member (did not identify herself)

A participant from the audience reminded us that there are many people involved in patient care: 2 million registered nurses, for example. Caregivers in many roles are users of electronic health records. We should be doing patient-centered and consumer-centered usability testing. We should be taking a team approach to usability testing. She suggests that AHRQ should focus on continuum of care instead of only ambulatory care and physicians.

Janey Barnes, User-View, Inc.

Vendors are doing user-centered design, but usability competes with other needs. She supports the idea that the government take the lead on

- Infrastructure to promote interoperability

- Funding and disseminating research

- Being an equal stakeholder with others

- Helping with education now! Because once people invest in an EHR, they aren't going to invest again

She believes that market forces will favor vendors who "get it" about usability, and that the government should allow those market forces to operate.

Charles Friedman, ONC

Dr. Friedman reminded workshop participants that the push to adoption is not a one-time event; it is ongoing. Even though the meaningful use rule for 2011 was announced today (July 13, 2010), work is already starting on Meaningful Use 2013. Work is also starting on what the next set of requirements for certification should be. He asked attendees: What should be in these future meaningful use policies?

Ross Koppel, University of Pennsylvania

Social innovations could be applied soon. In his recent studies of seven countries, if there was a national drug-drug integration database, drug-disease database, it sped up the system. Hospitals spend too much time individually updating formulary and barcodes. This is a waste of time. It could be improved.

Charles Webster, Encounter Pro, (audience)

What about the potential of free and open source EMR software? Could you discuss the safety side of using free open source EMR software?

Charles Goldsmith, Microsoft

The Common User Interface that he discussed in his talk is available.

Matthew Quinn, AHRQ

What gets overlooked in talking about open source is that it's not just a matter of free code, it's about communities. Communities need to form around open source software. People need to be given a choice to use a vendor interface or an open source vendor (plug and play). Open source has to involve both IT people and people with healthcare domain knowledge. What does the community do when domain changes mean changes to the software?

Svetlana Lowry, NIST

There is a preconceived notion regarding open source software that it is more usable because it has more input from end users. But there isn't a direct correlation between these two factors.

Walter Suarez, Head of Health IT for Kaiser Permanente, (audience)

Recommendation 1: The Stage 1 of Meaningful Use announced today included little about usability. He would like to take Meaningful Use a step further and propose a new concept called "*Meaningful Usability*." That would involve:

- Minimum standards of usability expected to be part of EHR

- Minimum set of certification criteria of functional usability capabilities

- Meaningful applicability of those standards in a real-life tool

Recommendation 2: He would then like the government to convene hearings to provide feedback to an advisory committee. These hearings would be held jointly to hear testimonies of what criteria should be recommended for standards and certification.

Recommendation 3: By Stage 2 of Meaningful Use, incorporate meaningful usability requirements. Usability would become mainstream, as it is not today.

Charles Friedman, ONC

This lays down a challenge that usability be measureable. If we are going to rise to the challenge that Dr. Suarez raised, we can't duck the measurability aspect of usability.

David Baquis, U.S. Access Board

Mr. Baquis would like to have accessibility discussed at one of the hearings that Dr. Suarez mentioned. He urges that whoever holds hearings make sure that the disability community knows about the hearings, has an opportunity to participate in the hearings, and be represented on any boards or groups that are looking into issues of meaningful usability.

Rebecca Grayson, User Reflections

Meaningful use requires usability. Tie them together into one concept.

Mary Crimmons, Apt Associates (audience)

Two comments:

- The federal government should come up with a comprehensive research agenda on all the topics we've discussed today that would be across agencies.

- She is optimistic that NIST will be able to test usability as they have been able to test other things.

Matthew Quinn, AHRQ

Mr. Quinn points out that a recent report from an expert panel that AHRQ put together includes research recommendations and policy recommendations. See http://healthit.ahrq.gov/portal/server.pt/gateway/PTARGS_0_11699_911984_0_0_18/EHRVendorPractices&Perspectives.pdf

David Baquis, U.S. Access Board

The Interagency Committee on Disability Research (ICDR) helps set the federal agenda for disability research. A report from the Committee goes to Congress and the President every year. Mr. Baquis said he would recommend to the Committee that a link to the proceedings of this workshop be distributed to the ICDR so they are aware of these issues.

Rob Kolodner, Open Health Tools, (audience)

With regard to the role of the government relative to the private sector:

In his previous experience, it took a long time to build accessibility into products and in some ways could not be accomplished because of how the tools had been built. So if the government is going to require this, let vendors know early so they can start working on the accessibility aspect of EHRs.

Why is the market not pushing this? Because the market is still immature and vendors drive the market.

Government needs to do things in the public's best interest. Could anything be done like SNOMED CT, which was so important it was bought into the public sector.

(Editor's note: SNOMED CT stands for Systematized Nomenclature of Medicine-Clinical Terms. Its web site says it "is considered to be the most comprehensive, multilingual clinical healthcare terminology in the world.")

Matthew Quinn, AHRQ

The report that the Altarum Institute recently completed was the first to talk to vendors (nine of them) about their processes.

Open source and communities around open source would open the market.

Another recommendation is to find a way to have a shared minimum data set for comparison rather than require vendors to hard code measures, which is going to take time to make it happen and to test it.

Jacob Reider, Allscripts

To report on stuff well, you have to describe it in systems the same way. Vocabularies exist out there.

SNOMED CT will be an important part of the EHR of tomorrow. What about interface terms? Which terms should we use? Should we impose words on our clinicians or let them tell us what the words should be?

Scott Lind, Siemens

The government should set a floor. Vendors should take usability as a baseline. The question is what level of usability is appropriate for an organization?

Charles Friedman, ONC

Dr. Friedman clarified what Lind was saying: Government's role is to establish a floor, a baseline – to set a minimum level for usability in systems. None of this prevents market innovation from vendors or makers of plug-ins or whatever, from going above and beyond – from reaching for the moon

Ross Koppel, University of Pennsylvania

Insurance companies are charging higher premiums to hospitals with EMRs, not because patients are worse off in such hospitals, but because the cost of forensic investigation is greater. With paper, you can find out easily who signed off on what when, but that's hard to do with an EMR.

Bob Schumacher, User Centric, (audience)

One way to drive the market is to get people who are purchasing to want something different. He did an analysis of 60 publicly available RFPs for EMRs. They don't mention usability. Buyers don't know how to think about usability. So the government could help by giving purchasers language for RFPs to buy a system with usability. Help purchasers write RFPs with the right questions to enable them to differentiate the usability of two different systems.

Svetlana Lowry, NIST

NIST has standards for user requirements that are publicly available. That they are not in RFPs is a shame.

David Baquis, U.S. Access Board

The government has a web site, www.buyaccessible.gov, which is specifically set up to help federal agencies buy accessible IT, including health IT. He tells a story of a vendor responding to a VA RFP that requires accessibility in its request for kiosks. The government takes the lead like this and it spills over to the private sector.

Vendors can voluntarily list themselves and describe the accessibility of their products. When government purchasers are looking for products, they would then find those vendors in the list.

Edna Boone, HIMSS

HIMSS is going to release a draft next week that will tell purchasers what sorts of questions to ask. It will be a draft because they hope to get feedback and additional resources.

MaryAnne Sterling, Sterling Health IT Consulting, (audience)

We need a good strategy and a press campaign for usability. Perhaps the government can help with that.

Appendix A:
Final Agenda

Usability in Health IT: Technical Strategy, Research, and Implementation

July 13, 2010

National Institute of Standards and Technology

Gaithersburg, MD

Final Agenda

8:00– 9:00 **Registration / Continental Breakfast**

9:00– 9:15 **Opening Remarks by ONC / NIST / AHRQ**

Farzad Mostashari, M.D., M.P.H., (Was unable to attend the workshop. Was represented by Charles P. Friedman, Chief Scientific Officer, ONC.)

Senior Advisor, ONC/HHS

Cita M. Furlani

Director, Information Technology Laboratory, NIST

9:15– 9:35 **Why are Electronic Health Records Hard to Use?**

The Good, the Bad, and the Ugly: Implementing an Electronic Health Record in an Innovative Medical Home Practice

Neil Patel, M.D.,

Associate Medical Director, Special Care Center

9:35– 10:30   **Current State of EHRs and Need for Action**

Meaningful Use: Meaning More? Or Meaning Less? Defining and Defying Sub-Clinical HIT

Ross Koppel, Ph.D.,

Professor, University of Pennsylvania

Best Practices in Usability and Information Design of Electronic Health Records

Kristen Werner, M.H.S.A.,

Senior Analyst, Altarum Institute

Presenting the EHR within the Provider and Patient's Digital Lifestyle

Clifford Goldsmith, M.D.,

Health Plan Industry Strategist, Microsoft Corporation

Usability, User Experience, and Clinician Happiness: What's the Connection

Jacob Reider, M.D.,

Chief Medical Informatics Officer, Allscripts

Usability Perspective from HIMSS

Edna Boone, M.A., C.P.H.I.M.S.,

Senior Director, Health Information Systems, HIMSS

Building Usability into Purchasing and Implementation Processes

Rebecca Grayson

Healthcare IT Usability Consultant and Principle, User Reflections

10:30 – 10:45   Coffee Break

10:45 – 11:45   Measuring and Reporting Usability

Methods of Measuring Usability

Charles P. Friedman, Ph.D.,

Chief Scientific Officer, ONC

Health IT Design and Usability : Myths and Realities

Bentzi Karsh, Ph.D.,

Associate Professor, University of Wisconsin

Evidence-Based Usability Practice

Kai Zheng, Ph.D.,

Assistant Professor, University of Michigan

Methods of Measuring Usability

Scott Lind

Director, User Experience, Soarian, Siemens Healthcare

Impacting Usability with Appropriate User-Based Research

Janey Barnes, Ph.D.,

Human Factors Specialist, User-View, Inc.

Usability Testing at CCHIT

Alisa Ray, M.S.,

Executive Director, CCHIT

11:45 – 12:30   **Points of Pain" – Addressing EHR User Disparities**

Accessibility and HIT

David Baquis

Accessibility Specialist, U.S. Access Board

Creating an Inclusive Infrastructure to Allow Affordable Access across Technologies, Disabilities and Ages

Gregg Vanderheiden, Ph.D.,

Professor and Director, Trace R&D Center,

University of Wisconsin

The SHARP Approach to EHR Usability

Jiajie Zhang, Ph.D.,

Dr. Doris L. Ross Professor and Associate Dean of Research,

University of Texas Health Science Center

TeachEHR: Who's Training the Clinical Workforce

Juan Gilbert, Ph.D.,

Professor and Chair of Human Centered Computing Division,

Clemson University

Usability is More than User Satisfaction: 10 Principles of EMR Usability

Jeffery Belden, M.D.,

Family Physician, University of Missouri

12:30 – 1:30   Lunch (NIST Cafeteria)

1:30 – 2:00   **Defining Federal Strategy: ONC, NIST, AHRQ, and FDA Usability Collective Efforts**

Building a Technical Framework for Usability and Accessibility of EHRs

Lana Lowry, Ph.D.,

Human Factors Lead, Health IT, NIST

AHRQ Research Efforts to Assess and Improve the Usability of EHRs

Matt Quinn, M.B.A.,

Special Expert, Health IT, AHRQ/HHS

Enhancing User Performance and Avoiding Safety Problems through Analysis, Discovery, Prioritization, and Design

Ron Kaye, M.A.,

Human Factors and Device Use-Safety Team Leader, FDA/HHS

2:00 – 3:00   **Recommendations and Next Steps**

Federal and Private Strategy and Tactics in Health IT Usability

All Roundtable and Audience Participants

Moderator: **Janice (Ginny) Redish, Ph.D.**

Discussion Points

- What should be the role of the federal government in improving the usability of EHRs?
- How can the federal government work to improve the availability of objective information about the usability of electronic health records?
- Based on the day's presentations, what are the key breakthroughs necessary to advance the usability of electronic health records? How can the federal government facilitate these breakthroughs?
- What are the key needs of the private sector efforts to improve usability that the government can support?

3:00 – 3:15   Coffee Break

3:15 – 4:45   Recommendations and Next Steps (Continued)

Appendix B:
List of Invited Workshop Participants

Roundtable Discussion Participants List

Last Name	First Name	Organization	Type
Baquis	David	U.S. Access Board	Government
Barnes	Janey	User-View, Inc.	Industry
Bean	Carol	ONC	Government
Belden	Jeffery	University of Missouri	Academia
Boone	Edna	HIMSS	Industry
Friedman	Charles	ONC	Government
Gilbert	Juan	Clemson University	Academia
Goldsmith	Clifford	Microsoft	Industry
Grayson	Rebecca	User Reflections	Industry
Jain	Sachin	ONC	Government
Karsh	Ben-Tzion	University of Wisconsin	Academia
Kaye	Ron	FDA	Government
Koppel	Ross	University of Pennsylvania	Academia
Lide	Bettijoyce	NIST	Government
Lind	Scott	Siemens Healthcare	Industry
Lowry	Lana	NIST	Government
Patel	Bakul	FDA	Government
Patel	Neil	Special Care Center	Industry/Healthcare
Quinn	Matt	AHRQ	Government
Ray	Alisa	CCHIT	Industry
Reider	Jacob	Allscripts	Industry
Shuren	Jeff	FDA	Government
Vanderheiden	Gregg	University of Wisconsin	Academia
Werner	Kristen	Altarum	Academia
Zayas-Caban	Teresa	AHRQ	Government
Zhang	Jiajie	University of Texas	Academia
Zheng	Kai	University of Michigan	Academia

Appendix C:
Speakers' Biographies

Health IT Usability Workshop

Biography of Roundtable Participants

David Baquis

Accessibility Specialist

U.S. Access Board

David Baquis is an Accessibility Specialist with the U.S. Access Board. He is currently leading a new rulemaking project to develop accessibility standards for medical diagnostic equipment, under authority of the recent healthcare reform law. He is also involved with updating accessibility standards and guidelines for information and communications technology under Section 508 of the Rehabilitation Act and Section 255 of the Telecommunications Act. Mr. Baquis writes technical assistance materials and has published many articles on assistive and accessible technology. In addition to responding to public inquiries, he delivers training including recent presentations on accessibility of: voting systems, e-learning, and health information technology. His background blends 30 years of experience in healthcare, consumer education, disability issues, technology, and public policy. Prior to his appointment at the Access Board, he worked as Director of the National Center on Hearing Assistive Technology.

Janey Barnes, Ph.D.,

Human Factors Specialist

User-View, Inc.

Janey Barnes currently is the principal of User-View, Inc. She has 15 plus years of experience as a Human Factors consultant serving diverse domains including healthcare, transportation, telecommunications, and financial sectors. She also has User-centered design experience with multiple hospital, ambulatory Electronic Medical Records (EMRs) and patient health portals. A current member of Healthcare Information and Management Systems Society (HIMSS), HFES, and Triangle Usability Professionals Association (UPA), she has a PhD in Cognitive Psychology.

Carol Bean, Ph.D., M.L.S., M.P.H.,

Director, Certification Division

Office of the National Coordinator for Health IT

Dr. Bean is currently Director of Certification at the Office of the National Coordinator for Health IT, where she leads activities related to testing and certification of EHR technology. She joined ONC in October 2007 to lead the standards harmonization program. Previously Dr. Bean served at the NIH in a variety of capacities over the past dozen years. She was a research scientist at the National Library of Medicine (NLM) and a program manager for biomedical informatics research and training at the NLM and at the National Center for Research Resources. Prior to joining ONC, Dr. Bean served as Chief Terminology Officer for the National Heart Lung and Blood Institute, where she coordinated Institute- and NIH-wide initiatives in interoperable data and terminology standards.

Dr. Bean did her doctoral work in psychology at the University of Georgia. She has Master's degrees in epidemiology, information science, and medical informatics; and completed postdoctoral fellowships in behavioral epidemiology at UC-Berkeley and in medical informatics at Columbia University. Her formal research interests address knowledge representation and conceptual structures, with special interest in semantic relationships.

Jeffery Belden, M.D.,

Associate Professor of Clinical Family & Community Medicine

University of Missouri-Columbia

Jeff Belden MD is a family physician on the faculty at the University of Missouri – Columbia in the Department of Family and Community Medicine, and on the affiliated faculty at the Information Experience Lab. He has a special interest in improving Electronic Health Record (EHR) usability, and in the visual display of information. Responsibilities currently include user training, implementations, collaboration in product development with Cerner on their ambulatory EHR, and collaboration with human-computer interaction colleagues in the IE Lab. He serves as Chair of the Healthcare Information and Management Systems Society (HIMSS) EMR Usability Task Force. His past experiences in photography, film-making, layout and design, typography, and consulting in healthcare software design inform his approach to user-centered design.

Edna Boone, M.A., C.P.H.I.M.S.,

Senior Director, Healthcare Information Systems

HIMSS

Edna Boone, MA, CPHIMS is Senior Director, Healthcare Information Systems, for the Healthcare Information and Management Systems Society (HIMSS), the largest U.S. not-for-profit healthcare association focused on providing global leadership for the optimal use of information technology. HIMSS represents approximately 23,000 individual members, more than 380 corporate members and nearly 30 not-for-profit organizations that share its mission.

She joined HIMSS in 2008 to oversee the Enterprise Information Systems Committee and Management Engineering – Process Improvement (ME-PI) Community for the Society working with HIMSS volunteers and industry leaders in these areas. In this position, Boone works with staff and member content experts to develop content materials including whitepapers, brochures, web content, and other resources and tools focused to educate the industry on Enterprise EHR and ME-PI issues such as EHR Adoption-Change Management, EHR Usability and Health IT Legal Aspects of the healthcare enterprise.

She also oversees the Grants Advantage program which provides education and a subscription service for HIMSS members which tracks funding opportunities for health information technology initiatives.

With more than 25 years experience in healthcare management, her career has focused on financial and clinical systems integration in ambulatory, acute and community care settings. She has extensive experience working with clinicians and served as Director of Clinical Systems and Physician Relations at United Health Services. She was also involved in the funding and development of the Southern Tier Health Link, a health information exchange covering seven counties in central New York, receiving 3.8 million dollars in start-up funds from the State of New York.

Boone has served as a Director in the Business Development department for Nextgen Healthcare systems focusing on health information technology grants and funding assistance for providers and health systems. She served HIMSS as a member of the Government Relations Roundtable and the Advocacy & Public Policy Steering Committee in 2007-2008.

She previously served as the president of MEDIA Medical Education and Information Association and as an active member of New York Medical Group Management Association (NYMGMA). In addition, she received several community and organizational awards for leadership.

A native of New Jersey, Boone has a BS degree in Marketing from Michigan State University and a MS degree in Social Science with a focus on Medical Informatics, from the State University of New York, Binghamton. She currently lives on Capital Hill in Washington, DC and works in the HIMSS Arlington, Virginia office.

Charles Friedman, Ph.D.,

Chief Scientific Officer

Office of the National Coordinator for Health IT

Charles P. Friedman, PhD. is currently the Chief Scientific Officer for the Office of the National Coordinator for Health Information Technology (ONC) in the U.S. Department of Health and Human Services (HHS). As ONC's chief scientist, he leads a group responsible for tracking and promoting innovation in health IT, for research programs to improve technology, for applications of health IT that support basic and clinical research, for evaluation of all of ONC's programs, for programs to develop the health IT workforce, and for activities supporting global eHealth. Dr. Friedman served as Deputy National Coordinator for two years prior to assuming his new position. He was lead author of the national Health IT Strategic Plan released in June of 2008.

Prior to joining ONC, Dr. Friedman was Associate Director of the National Heart, Lung, and Blood Institute of the National Institutes of Health (NIH). In this capacity, he founded the Center for Research Informatics and Information Technology, and functioned as the Institute's Chief Information Officer. Dr. Friedman first joined NIH in 2003, as a Senior Scholar at the National Library of Medicine.

From 1996 to 2003, Dr. Friedman was Professor and Associate Vice Chancellor for Biomedical Informatics at the University of Pittsburgh where he established a health sciences-wide Center for Biomedical Informatics, a well-funded program of informatics research, and masters and doctoral degree programs in biomedical informatics. He also served as Chief Information Officer for the University of Pittsburgh Schools of the Health Sciences.

Dr. Friedman obtained bachelors and masters degrees in physics from the Massachusetts Institute of Technology (MIT) and also received a PhD in education from the University of North Carolina (UNC).

He wrote his first computer program in 1966. He spent over 19 years on the medical school faculty at UNC and served as Assistant Dean for Medical Education and Informatics. In 1985, he established the Laboratory for Computing and Cognition at UNC and, in 1992, started UNC's medical informatics training program.

Dr. Friedman has written extensively for scientific journals, and authored a well-known textbook. He is a past president of the American College of Medical Informatics, and was the 2005 chair of the Annual Symposium of the American Medical Informatics Association. He currently serves as Associate Editor of the Journal of the American Medical Informatics Association.

Juan Gilbert, Ph.D.,

Professor and Chair, Human Centered Computing Division

Clemson University

Dr. Juan E. Gilbert is a Professor and Chair of the Human Centered Computing Division in the School of Computing at Clemson University where he leads the Interaction and Information Lab. Dr. Gilbert has research projects in spoken language systems, advanced learning technologies, usability and accessibility, Ethnocomputing (Culturally Relevant Computing) and databases/data mining. He has published more than 100 articles, given more than 150 talks and obtained more than $12 million dollars in research funding. He was recently named one of the 50 most important African-Americans in Technology. He was also named a Speech Technology Luminary by Speech Technology Magazine and a national role model by Minority Access Inc. Dr. Gilbert is also a National Associate of the National Research Council of the National Academies, an ACM Distinguished Speaker and a Senior Member of the Institute of Electrical and Electronics Engineers (IEEE) Computer Society. Recently, Dr. Gilbert was named a Master of Innovation by Black Enterprise Magazine, a Modern-Day Technology Leader by the Black Engineer of the Year Award Conference, the Pioneer of the Year by the National Society of Black Engineers and he received the Black Data Processing Association (BDPA) Epsilon Award for Outstanding Technical Contribution. In 2002, Dr. Gilbert was named one of the nation's top African-American Scholars by Diverse Issues in Higher Education. Dr. Gilbert recently testified before the Congress on the Bipartisan Electronic Voting Reform Act of 2008 for his innovative work in electronic voting. He is a Fellow in the Center for Governmental Services at Auburn University as well. In 2006, Dr. Gilbert was honored with a mural painting in New York City by City Year New York, a non-profit organization that unites a diverse group of 17 to 24 year-old young people for a year of full-time, rigorous community service, leadership development, and civic engagement.

Clifford Goldsmith, M.D.,

Health Plan Solutions Strategist

Microsoft Corporation

Clifford Goldsmith MD, a Microsoft Solution Strategist for the US, provides strategic expertise to Health Plans. Dr. Goldsmith brings a unique experience to Microsoft as a physician who also has over 25 years of know-how envisioning, designing, developing, and selling high-performance technology solutions for the healthcare industry.

Dr. Goldsmith has worked for Microsoft Corporation for over 10 years, serving in several roles including a Managing Consultant in MCS and the US Director for the Provider Industry. He focused on numerous areas of health IT including clinical collaboration, pharmaceutical clinical trials, medical devices and embedded systems, agents for home care, as well as Microsoft's Physician Digital Dashboard and Clinical Portals. Dr. Goldsmith helped Microsoft executives set strategic direction for the healthcare investments.

Dr. Goldsmith was also Chief Medical Officer of Aptima Corporation, where he led a team in transitioning well-tested concepts on human-centered engineering from aviation and the military into healthcare. He was the co-founder of LINK Medical Computing, which produces a commercial product for integrating medical devices with Hospital Information Systems. Before LINK, he worked for Harvard University's Department of Medicine and the Center for Clinical Computing, developing and managing various aspects of the HIS for both Beth Israel and Brigham and Women's Hospitals. During this appointment, he pioneered full, remote access electrocardiograph (ECG) integration HIS and implemented it at the Beth Israel Hospital. He was a founding member of Microsoft Healthcare Users Group (MSHUG) and joined the HL7 (Health Level 7) Committee in its early years. Dr. Goldsmith received a B.S. and a M.D. from the University of Witwatersrand, South Africa. He has practiced clinical medicine and also worked for the National Center for Occupational Healthcare, Division of Epidemiology, Johannesburg, South Africa, where he designed, developed and supported software for clinical research, including pulmonary function and surgical pathology databases.

Dr Goldsmith has actively participated in Massachusetts health initiatives including the Massachusetts Regional Health Information Organization (RHIO) and the recent efforts on affordable, available health insurance.

Rebecca Grayson

Healthcare IT Usability Consultant and Principle

User Reflections

Rebecca Grayson is an independent Health IT consultant with over 20 years experience in the design, usability and implementation of Electronic Medical Records (EMRs). She served as Usability and Design Manager in the development of an EMR for a teaching hospital with distributed ambulatory care centers and a regional hospital network (Marquette General Health System and Kaiser Permanente). She has extensive experience working with clinical end-users from requirements and design through implementations, with specialized expertise in ambulatory care systems, clinical documentation tools and software usability. Rebecca holds a Computer Science degree from San Francisco State University as well as graduate education in Medical Informatics at UCSF and a Human Factors degree from the University of Idaho.

Sachin Jain, M.D., M.B.A.,

Special Assistant to the National Coordinator

Office of the National Coordinator for Health IT

Sachin H. Jain is special assistant to the National Coordinator for Health Information Technology in the Obama Administration. In this role, he works closely with Dr. Blumenthal in executing his health IT agenda, leading initiatives on usability, private sector engagement, and disparities in care. Prior to joining the administration, he was a member of the faculty at Harvard Business School and a resident physician at the Brigham and Women's Hospital.

Dr. Jain holds his bachelor's degree (AB), medical degree (MD), and MBA from Harvard University. A Paul and Daisy Soros Fellow, Dr. Jain has worked previously at McKinsey and Co, WellPoint, and the Institute for Healthcare Improvement. He was principal investigator on three Commonwealth Fund grants used to found and support ImproveHealthCare.org, an organization that aims to educate physicians about health care systems. He has served as a guest instructor at the MIT-Sloan School of Management, and the Darden School at the University of Virginia.

While he was faculty at the Institute for Strategy and Competitiveness at Harvard Business School, Dr. Jain worked closely with strategy professor Michael Porter on research into health care delivery reform.

He was a founding member and associate director of the Global Health Delivery Project housed at the Institute and Harvard Medical School and has consulted widely across the health care sector, including for several small health information technology companies.

Dr. Jain's writings have appeared in The New England Journal of Medicine, Health Affairs and other publications. The book he co-edited (with Susan Pories and Gordon Harper) The Soul of A Doctor (Algonquin Press: Chapel Hill) was published in 2006 and has been translated into Chinese (2008).

A native of Bergen County, NJ, Dr. Jain now resides in Washington, DC.

Ben-Tzion Karsh, Ph.D.,

Associate Professor, Industrial and Systems Engineering,

University of Wisconsin-Madison

Ben-Tzion (Bentzi) Karsh, PhD, is an Associate Professor of Industrial and Systems Engineering at the University of Wisconsin-Madison where his specialty is human factors engineering. He has secondary appointments in the departments of Family Medicine, Population Health, and Biomedical Engineering at the University of Wisconsin and the Department of Health Administration at Virginia Commonwealth University. His research, which has been funded by the Agency for Healthcare Research and Quality (AHRQ), United Kingdom Department of Health, Robert Woods Johnson Foundation, and the National Library of Medicine, focuses on using human factors engineering methods to study and improve pediatric inpatient and elderly primary care patient safety. His studies focus on understanding the complex interactions among clinicians, the artifacts they use, and the contexts in which they work.

Dr. Karsh has authored or co-authored over 100 journal articles, conference papers and book chapters. His most recent publications focus on interruptions in healthcare, violations of medication safety protocols, health information technology design and implementation, nursing mental workload, and the design of consumer health informatics. He has served as an expert panelist on several invited panels and workshops sponsored by AHRQ and the Office of the National Coordinator (ONC) on topics related to consumer and clinician decision support.

He is a past national Chair of the Health Care Technical Group of the Human Factors and Ergonomics Society, serves as an ad hoc study section member for AHRQ, and is a peer reviewer for journals such as the British Medical Journal, Joint Commission Journal on Quality and Safety, Quality and Safety in Healthcare, (Journal of the American Medical Informatics Association (JAMIA), Annals of Emergency Medicine, Annals of Family Medicine, Behavior and Information Technology, Applied Ergonomics and Human Factors. Dr. Karsh has co-directed a professional short course for the last six years that has trained nearly 200 clinicians, health administrators, and patient safety leaders in the application of human factors engineering methods and tools for patient safety.

Ron Kaye, M.A.,

Team Leader, Human Factors and Device Use-Safety Office of Device Evaluation

Center for Devices and Radiological Health, U.S. Food and Drug Administration

Mr. Kaye represents the Human Factors program at the Food and Drug Administration (FDA's) Center for Devices and Radiological Health. He leads the Human Factors and Device Use Safety group which is located in the CDRH Office of Device Evaluation (ODE). The purpose of the FDA's Human Factors program is to ensure that new medical devices are safe and effective when used by the intended population of users. The primarily effort involves reviewing new device submissions, promoting effective and focused human factors evaluation and good design practices for medical devices, development of FDA's Human Factors Guidance, and participation with National and International Human Factors Standards. The team also contributes to analysis of post-market reports of use-related error and device recalls where use error is involved.

Ron has a BS degree in Psychology and Biology, and a MA in Applied Psychology. He has worked in Human Factors for 27 years and has been with FDA's Center for Devices and Radiological Health (CDRH) for 14 years. Prior to joining the FDA, Ron worked with Human Factors and human performance testing, training analysis, and research on safety-critical systems such as nuclear power plant control rooms, military weapons and communications systems, aircraft cockpit systems, air traffic control systems, and medical devices.

Ross Koppel, Ph.D.,

Faculty, Sociology Department,

University of Pennsylvania

Professor Ross Koppel's work in medical informatics reflects his 40 year career as researcher and professor of sociology of work and organizations, statistics, ethnographic research, survey research, and medical sociology. He is the principal investigator of University of Pennsylvania's study on hospital workplace culture and medication errors. In the past 4 years Dr. Koppel has published over 25 articles and book chapters on health IT in the Journal of the American Medical Association (JAMA), Health Affairs, Journal of the American Medical informatics Association (JAMIA), Journal of Biomedical Informatics, Journal of Clinical Care, Journal of the American Geriatrics Society, Journal of Managed Care, Agency for Healthcare Research and Quality (AHRQ), and Infection Control and Hospital Epidemiology plus two books (one on research methods (Sage Publications) and one in press). Koppel is also the author of several works on evaluation and use of statistical methods in medical settings.

His work generally combines sophisticated statistical analyses with survey research and skilled ethnographic research—focusing on use of health IT *in situ*. Professor Koppel is currently co Principal Investigator (PI) of an AHRQ-funded project to develop a guide to implementing health IT while mitigating unintended consequences. That guide is based on new models of interactions between technology and organizations, which Koppel co-authored with Michael Harrison. In addition to his work in medical informatics, Koppel has authored over a 160 academic papers and articles, several monographs, and several books and book chapters. Many of those works addressed the interaction between technology and the workplace, training for use of technology, hospitals as workplaces, illness and society, and the cost of disease and care giving to the U. S. economy.

Dr. Koppel is the recipient of the Distinguished Career Award in the Practice of Sociology from the American Sociological Association (ASA). He has also been honored with the William Foote Whyte Award from the ASA's section on Public Sociology, the Robert E. Park Award from the Association for Applied and Clinical Sociology, the Distinguished Career Award from the Society for Applied Sociology, and several other awards for his work in Sociological scholarship and practice. He has served as president of all of America's associations of applied sociologists. Koppel also is the incoming chair of AMIA's Evaluation Working Group, sits on several academic journal editorial boards, serves on the Board of the European Sociology Association's Section on Qualitative Methods, has twice served on the White House Conference on Future of Small Business & Entrepreneurship, was president of the section on Temporal Ecology of the Research Committee on Social Ecology of the International Sociological Association, and has served as an evaluator for the National Science Foundation, the National Endowment for the Humanities, and the Agency for Healthcare Research and Quality (AHRQ).

Many of Professor Koppel's writing in medical informatics are considered classics in the field.

Bettijoyce Lide, M.S.,

Senior Advisor and Program Coordinator for Health IT

National Institute of Standards and Technology

Bettijoyce Lide is the Senior Advisor and Program Coordinator for health IT in NIST's Information Technology Laboratory. She serves as program lead for NIST's health IT responsibilities outlined in the American Recovery and Reinvestment Act (ARRA) and for the NIST-Department of Health and Human Services (HHS)/Office of the National Coordinator for Health Information Technology (ONC) collaboration. She leads a NIST team in a broad range of initiatives to help enable the majority of Americans to have electronic health records and the development of a nationwide health information network by 2014.

Prior to that, Bettijoyce Lide was with the Advanced Technology Program (ATP), serving as both Competitions Manager and Program Manager, designing, implementing, and managing the Information Infrastructure for Healthcare Program. Earlier, she served as Scientist, Programmer, and Group Leader of the Data Systems Development Group, Standard Reference Data, leading cutting-edge applications of computer technology to the storage, analysis, retrieval, and dissemination of evaluated chemical and physical data.

Scott Lind

Director, User Experience, Soarian

Siemens Healthcare

Scott Lind has been leading User Experience teams for the past 12 years in the design of web and mobile applications. Before joining Siemens Healthcare in 2005, he was Director of Usability Engineering at Telcordia Technologies (formerly part of Bell Labs).

Lana Lowry

Human Factors Lead for Health Care IT

National Institute of Standards and Technology

Lana Lowry is NIST's expert and project lead on usability for health IT. Lana has conducted extensive applied research in usability and accessibility for several government agencies, most recently on voting systems in the United States for the National Institute of Standards and Technology (NIST). The goal of her research is to improve systems by developing usability and accessibility standards and testing protocols for laboratories to apply to the certification of the systems. Lana has published and presented extensively in the areas of human factors and ergonomics worldwide. Her expertise is in the design of complex systems and software for mission-critical and real-time environments; in the application of human reliability analysis and human error analysis to complex human-machine interactions in automated systems and software; and in the development of standards and methods for evaluating, testing, and improving system and application interfaces.

Lana served as a senior research scientist on a program providing human factors for the Earth Observing System Data and Information System (EOSDIS) Core System, part of the National Aeronautics and Space Administration's (NASA) Mission to Planet Earth. Later on, at NCR Corporation's Government Systems Division, Lana led a team of usability engineers for ten years, applying her knowledge and expertise in HCI and usability through product innovation in the retail markets, e-commerce solutions, and government systems environments.

Bakul Patel, M.S., M.B.A.,

Policy Advisor, Office of Center Director,

Center for Devices and Radiological Health, U.S. Food and Drug Administration

Bakul Patel currently holds the position of Policy Advisor in the Office of Center Director, Center for Devices and Radiological Health (CDRA), FDA. In this position, Mr. Patel is responsible for leading several efforts related to CDRH's policy on medical device software and systems. Mr. Patel is also responsible for advising the Center Director on regulatory issues related to health information technology and mHealth. Mr. Patel started at FDA in CDRH, Office of Compliance as a Compliance Officer. Prior to joining FDA, Mr. Patel was a senior consultant with the USDA as a Lean Six Sigma Black Belt for the modernization project for farm services agency. Mr. Patel's previous experiences include working as Senior Program Manager at EMC Corp., where he developed software products for archiving and storage industry. He has held several positions since 1986 as a senior product manager, software engineering manager and as a software/systems engineer with various high technology organizations. Mr. Patel has also worked with fast paced, technology intensive organizations within the semiconductor capital equipment industry. Mr. Patel has a MS in Electrical Engineering from the University of Regina, Canada and a MBA from Johns Hopkins University, Baltimore.

Neil Patel, M.D.,

Associate Medical Director

Special Care Center

Neil Patel MD is Special Care's associate medical director. Born and raised in Piscataway, New Jersey, he is the son of Indian émigrés from the Gujarat area of northwestern India. Patel earned his medical degree at the New Jersey Medical School and trained in family medicine at Boston University. During his residency he took advantage of opportunities to work in primary and HIV care in Lesotho, Africa; in obstetrics in Guayaquil, Ecuador; and in inpatient surgical care in Vadodara, India. Patel's job at the Special Care Center is his first since completing his residency. Patel is fluent in Gujarati, the language spoken in and around Gujarat, thus able to communicate easily with some of the Indian immigrants enrolled at the Special Care Center—making them truly feel as if they have a real medical home in the United States.

Matthew Quinn, M.B.A.,

Special Expert, Health IT,

Center for Primary Care, Prevention, and Clinical Partnerships

Agency for Healthcare Research and Quality (AHRQ)

Matt Quinn is a Special Expert in the Agency for Healthcare Research and Quality (AHRQ) Healthcare IT group. Before joining AHRQ, Mr. Quinn was the Healthcare Program Manager for Teradata, the global leader in data warehousing and analytic technologies, and was responsible for healthcare strategy and partnerships for the company. Prior, he led marketing for Quantros, a patient safety and clinical outcomes improvement software company, managed GE Healthcare's "Six Sigma for Healthcare" clinical outcomes performance improvement consulting services and data analytic products, helped build an early Personal Health Record (PHR) company, and served as an Army Engineer Officer.

Matt's published work can be seen in a variety of healthcare and technology publications and journals, and he has spoken at the World Health Care Congress, eHealth Initiative's Health IT Summit, and other national and international venues.

Matt Quinn earned a BS from the United States Military Academy at West Point and an MBA from Colorado State University.

Alisa Ray

Executive Director

Certification Commission for Healthcare Information Technology (CCHIT)

Joining the Certification Commission for Healthcare Information Technology (CCHIT) in January 2006, as its first Executive Director, Ms Ray supports the work of CCHIT's Boards of Commissioners and Trustees and its Workgroups, manages CCHIT's business operations, and develops staff and resources. She has managed and executed the three year $7.5 million federal contract to develop certification criteria and inspection process. Ms. Ray has overseen the launch of CCHIT's EHR certification programs in the ambulatory and inpatient domains as well as expansion areas.

She was previously an Assistant Vice President of Certification and Information Products at the National Committee for Quality Assurance (NCQA), a private, non-profit organization dedicated to improving health care quality through the accreditation and certification of a wide range of health care organizations. During her tenure at NCQA, she guided the product development and launch of several new information products including the Healthcare Effectiveness Data and Information Set (HEDIS) Software Certification Program and the HEDIS Compliance Audit™. Formerly, as Senior Research Associate at the American Association of Health Plans, she managed initiatives in the areas of outcomes research, quality improvement and clinical performance measurement. At Medstat, she held product development, marketing and client consulting roles.

Ms. Ray received her Master's in Health Services Administration from the University of Michigan School of Public Health and BS in Psychology from the University of Michigan.

Jacob Reider, M.D.,

Chief Medical Informatics Officer

Allscripts

Jacob Reider is a family physician and Chief Medical Informatics Officer for Allscripts.

He has 15 years of experience in Healthcare Information Technology with special interest in user experience and information portability. He serves on the Executive Committee of the Healthcare Information and Management Systems Society (HIMSS) Electronic Health Records Association (EHRA) and as Chair of the EHRA Quality and Clinical Decision Support SIG, and Electronic Health Record Association (EHRA) Liaison to the HIMSS Clinical Decision Support Task Force. He serves on the Agency for Healthcare Research and Quality (AHRQ) Clinical Decision Support (CDS) Technical Expert Panel, and was a member of the National Quality Forum's Health Information Technology Expert Panel's (HITEP II) Quality Data Set Workgroup.

Jeff Shuren, M.D., J.D.,

Director, Center for Devices and Radiological Health,

U.S. Food and Drug Administration

Dr. Jeffrey E. Shuren is the Director of the Center for Devices and Radiological Health at the Food and Drug Administration (FDA). The Center is responsible for assuring the safety, effectiveness, and quality of medical devices, assuring the safety of radiation-emitting products (such as cell phones and microwaves), and fostering device innovation.

Dr. Shuren served as the Acting Deputy Commissioner for Policy, Planning, and Budget from August 2009 to September 2009, Associate Commissioner for Policy and Planning from March 2008 to August 2009, and Special Counsel to the Principal Deputy Commissioner from March 2009 to September 2009. From March 2003 to March 2008 Dr. Shuren was the Assistant Commissioner for Policy, and was the medical officer in the Office of Policy from 1998 to 2001. Dr. Shuren served as the Director of the Division of Items and Devices, Coverage and Analysis Group at the Centers for Medicare and Medicaid Services. From 1999-2000 he served as a detailee on the Senate Health, Education, Labor, and Pensions Committee. From 1998 to 2003 Dr. Shuren also was as a Staff Volunteer in the National Institutes of

Health's Cognitive Neuroscience Section where he supervised and designed clinical studies on human reasoning.

Dr. Shuren received his B.S. and M.D. degrees from Northwestern University under its Honors Program in Medical Education. He completed his medical internship at Beth Israel Hospital in Boston, his neurology residency at Tufts New England Medical Center, and a fellowship in behavioral neurology and neuropsychology at the University of Florida. He received his J.D. from the University of Michigan. Dr. Shuren joined the University of Cincinnati College of Medicine's Department of Neurology as an Assistant Professor where he led two active memory disorders clinics and implemented a research program in Alzheimer's disease and disorders of higher cognitive function.

Gregg Vanderheiden, Ph.D.,

Professor and Director, Trace R&D Center,

University of Wisconsin-Madison

Gregg Vanderheiden is a professor of Industrial and Biomedical Engineering, and director of Trace R&D Center at the University of Wisconsin-Madison. He has worked in technology and disability for more than 35 years and currently directs the National Institute on Disability and Rehabilitation Research (NIDRR) Rehabilitation Engineering Research Center (RERC) on Information Technology Access, and co-directs the RERC on Telecommunications Access (joint with Gallaudet University).

Dr. Vanderheiden was a pioneer in the field of Augmentative Communication (a term taken from his writings in 1979), and worked with people having physical, visual, hearing and cognitive disabilities. His work with the computer industry led to many of the access features that are standard today. For example, access features developed by Dr. Vanderheiden and his team (e.g., MouseKeys, etc.) have been built into the Macintosh OS since 1987, OS/2 and the UNIX X Window system since 1993, and more than half a dozen were built into Windows 95, 98, NT, 2000, XP, Vista and now System 7. His work is also found in the built-in access features in ATMs, Point of Sale terminals, and cross-disability accessible USPS Automated Postal Stations, as well as the accessible Amtrak ticket machines, and in airport terminals.

Dr. Vanderheiden has served on numerous professional, industry and government advisory and planning committees including those for the Federal Communications Commission (FCC), National Science Foundation (NSF), National Institutes of Health (NIH), Veterans Affairs (VA), General Service Administration (GSA), National Council on Disability (NCD), Access Board and White House. Dr. Vanderheiden served on the Federal Communications Commission (FCC's) Technological Advisory

Council, was a member of the Telecommunications Access Advisory committee and the Electronic Information Technology Access Advisory Committee (508 and 255 refresh) for the US Access Board, and served on the steering committee for the National Research Council's Planning Group on "Every Citizen Interfaces," and the National Academies' Institute of Medicine Committee on the Future of Disability in America.

He has received over 30 awards for his work on technology and disability include the ACM Social Impact Award for the Human-Computer Interaction Community, the Ron Mace Award, the Access award from AFB, the Yuri Rubinski Memorial World Wide Web Award (WWW6), and the Isabelle and Leonard H. Goldenson Award for Outstanding Research in Medicine and Technology (UCPA).

Kristen Werner, M.H.S.A.,

Senior Analyst

Altarum Institute

Kristen Werner, MHSA is a Senior Analyst at the Altarum Institute, specializing in projects that increase the value realized through the implementation of health IT. Through applying economic analysis, usability analysis, and cognitive task analysis, she supports organizations in the strategic and operational planning required for effective selection and use of health IT. Ms. Werner led the Agency for Healthcare Research and Quality (AHRQ) commissioned project on the "Use of Dense Display and Information Design Principles in Primary Care Health IT Systems." establishing a foundation of EHR user interface design considerations and the application of information design principles to the use of health IT in primary care settings and is currently exploring the use of Cognitive Task Analysis in supporting the implementation of clinical decision support systems.

Teresa Zayas-Caban, Ph.D.,

Senior Manager for Health IT

Agency for Healthcare Research and Quality (AHRQ)

Teresa Zayas Cabán, Ph.D., serves as senior manager for health information technology (health IT) at the Agency for Healthcare Research and Quality (AHRQ). She oversees projects in the portfolio implementing and demonstrating the value of health IT. Dr. Zayas Cabán leads the Enabling Patient-Centered Care through Health IT grant initiative. She also manages several contracts focused on clinical decision support, workflow, and on the design and implementation of health IT and its impact to consumers.

Dr. Zayas Cabán completed her doctoral training at the University of Wisconsin-Madison where she was a National Science Foundation Graduate Research Fellow in industrial engineering. Her dissertation work focused on the development of a methodology that captures the location and distribution of health information in the home. Before joining AHRQ, she served as a post-doctoral trainee in the Computation and Informatics in Biology and Medicine program in Wisconsin examining the informed-consent process for health research projects to discover factors that influence the quality of decisions made by potential participants about whether or not to participate in a study.

Her interests include understanding how to apply human factors engineering concepts in the home environment, how to capture home health information management work, and access to care.

Jiajie Zhang, Ph.D.,

Dr. Doris L. Ross Professor & Associate Dean of Research

PI & Co-Director, National Center for Cognitive Informatics and Decision Making in Healthcare

University of Texas Health Science Center at Houston

Dr. Zhang is the Dr. Doris L. Ross Professor and has been the Associate Dean for Research since 2002 at the School of Health Information Sciences. He is a researcher, teacher, and administrator. As a researcher, he has spent the past two decades doing research in biomedical informatics, cognitive science, human-centered computing, decision making, and information visualization. He has authored more than 120 journal articles, book chapters, and peer-reviewed proceedings papers. He has been the principal investigator or co-investigator on more than two dozen grants from the Office of the National Coordinator (ONC), National Aeronautics and Space Administration (NASA), Office of Naval Research, Army, National Institutes of Health (NIH), James S. McDonnell Foundation, State of Texas, and other funding agencies. Most recently he is the Principal Investigator of a $15 million award for the National Center for Cognitive Informatics and Decision Making in Healthcare under ONC's SHARP program for Patient-Centered Cognitive Support. As a teacher, he has been teaching courses in human-computer interaction, information visualization, and technology-mediated social dynamics. He has supervised or co-supervised nearly twenty PhD students and over sixty master's students. Dr. Zhang was a recipient of John P. McGovern Outstanding Teacher Award. As the Associate Dean for Research he helped the school increase its research funding and expenditures at a fast rate. He was instrumental in establishing a few research centers: Center for Cognitive Informatics and Decision Making (Co-Director), Center for Translational Neuroinformatics (Acting Director), the Joint UTH-UTMB Center for Personalized Biomedical Informatics, and the newly ONC-funded National Center for Cognitive Informatics and Decision Making in Healthcare (Co-Director). Dr. Zhang also has some training in academic leadership and business administration. Dr. Zhang is an elected Fellow of American College of Medical Informatics.

Kai Zheng, Ph.D.,

Assistant Professor

Information Systems and Health Informatics

The University of Michigan

Kai Zheng is jointly appointed as Assistant Professor of Health Management and Policy in the School of Public Health, Assistant Professor of Information in the School of Information, and Adjunct Assistant Professor in the School of Nursing at the University of Michigan. He is also affiliated with the Medical School Center for Computational Medicine and Biology and the Michigan Institute for Clinical and Health Research. Zheng's research and teaching are in the area of information systems, particularly focusing on health informatics, which studies the use of information, communication, and decision technologies in healthcare delivery and management. His recent work investigates innovative technologies supporting medical knowledge management and clinical decision-making, and topics related to interaction design and workflow and sociotechnical integration.

Zheng holds a Ph.D. degree in Information Systems from Carnegie Mellon University, where his dissertation entitled "Design, Implementation, User Acceptance, and Evaluation of a Clinical Decision Support System for Evidence-Based Medicine Practice" received the 2007 William W. Cooper Doctoral Dissertation Award in Management or Management Sciences.

Ginny Redish, Ph.D., (Moderator)

President

Redish & Associates, Inc.

Dr. Janice (Ginny) Redish is President of Redish & Associates, Inc. in Bethesda, Maryland. For more than 30 years, Ginny has been helping clients through her expertise in user-centered design, usability, and clear communication. Ginny is co-author of two of the classic books on user-centered design (on usability testing and on user- and task analysis for interface design). Her most recent book, on writing great web content, received rave reviews and has been featured in many blogs, including ones that focus on health literacy.

Ginny is sought-after as a speaker, workshop leader, and facilitator. She has keynoted conferences in seven countries and has trained thousands of professionals in how to communicate clearly and how to create usable and useful systems.

Ginny's research covers a wide range of topics within the fields of usability, accessibility, and plain language. For the National Institute of Standards and Technology (NIST), her research on usability and language in ballots contributed to the development of the framework for voting standards. For the Department of Health and Human Services (HHS), she has studied how blind and low-vision users work with web sites. For American Association of Retired Persons (AARP), she developed a multi-faceted model of older adults that helps system designers and evaluators understand the diversity within our current population of seniors.

Appendix D:
Presentation Summaries

Health IT Usability Workshop

Presentation Summaries of Roundtable Participants

The Good, the Bad, and the Ugly: Implementing an Electronic Health Record in an Innovative Medical Home Practice

Neil Patel, M.D.,

Associate Medical Director

Special Care Center

The American Recovery and Reinvestment Act (ARRA) of 2009 will soon provide billions of dollars to small physician practices nationwide to encourage adoption of Electronic Health Records (EHRs). Although shifting from paper to computers should lead to better and cheaper care, the transition is complex. This presentation describes the struggles to adapt a commercial electronic health record to an innovative practice serving high-cost patients with chronic diseases. Limitations in the technology gave rise to medication errors, interruptions in work flow, and other problems common to paper systems. Our experience should encourage providers and policy makers to consider alternative software and informatics models before investing in currently available systems.

Meaningful Use: Meaning More? or Meaning Less? Defining and Defying Sub-Clinical Health IT

Ross Koppel, Ph.D.,

Faculty, Sociology Department,

University of Pennsylvania

This presentation briefly reviews:

- The motivation and rationale for meaningful use (MU) measures-examining the reasonable responsibilities of those receiving subsides and the MU marketing advantages for Health IT vendors
- The development of the MU measures
- Their appropriateness for care improvement
- Their value to the development of Health IT
- The role of certification systems (previous and current)
- The real and supposed barriers to Health IT implementation
- The controversy over timing

Best Practices in Usability and Information Design of Electronic Health Records (EHRs)

Kristen Werner, M.H.S.A.,

Senior Analyst

Altarum Institute

A recently completed Agency for Healthcare Research and Quality (AHRQ) study examined current vendor process for employing usability standards and "best practices" throughout the design and deployment of ambulatory Electronic Health Record (EHR) systems. While vendor interviews revealed a deep commitment to the creation of high quality usable products with end users consultation throughout the design and development process; formal usability testing is still fairly uncommon, and EHR specific standards and best practices are almost non-existent. Given current end user dissatisfaction with the ability to integrate existing Health IT solutions into clinical workflows and the role of government in subsidizing the purchase and use of EHRs, these findings present a challenging environment for those attempting to evaluate, promote or use Electronic Health Records (EHRs).

Presenting the Electronic Health Record (EHR) within the Provider and Patient's Digital Lifestyle

Clifford Goldsmith, M.D.,

Health Plan Solutions Strategist

Microsoft Corporation

Electronic Health Record (EHR) Meaningful Use is about improved quality and safety. It is clear that IT can achieve both these goals especially if we take advantage of new collaborative technologies and unified communications to engage the providers and patients across all components of their digital lifestyle. However, we need to ensure that introducing new technologies does not also introduce new medical errors. To avoid this trap we must have commonality in the clinical User Interface across channels, devices and modalities. In this short presentation we will discuss how Microsoft worked with the National Health Service (NHS) to set up clinical User Interface (UI) guidelines, create common controls and samples, work with software vendors to innovate within this extensible framework and thereby provider a safer, compelling clinical user environment.

Usability, User Experience, and Clinician Happiness: What's the Connection?

Jacob Reider, M.D.,

Chief Medical Informatics Officer

Allscripts

Usability, while long ignored in Health IT, is now the talk of the town. But are we raising the bar high enough? Do we want software to be functional, or could/should we aim beyond to make it pleasurable? How do we measure users' emotional responses to our products, and how can this inform future design?

Usability Perspective from HIMSS

Edna Boone, M.A., C.P.H.I.M.S.,

Senior Director, Healthcare Information Systems

Healthcare Information and Management System Society (HIMSS)

This presentation will include a review of current status hospital and health system Health IT deployment as well as potential education opportunities for disseminating usability basics critical in the configuration, customization and implementation stages. Planned HIMSS Electronic Health Record (EHR) Taskforce Deliverables for 2010-2011 will also be presented.

Building Usability into Purchasing and Implementation Processes

Rebecca Grayson

Healthcare IT Usability Consultant and Principle

User Reflections

Ms. Grayson thinks the academics and government members of the panel will provide sufficient coverage of the medium and long term strategies for improving the usability of Electronic Health Records (EHRs) (standards, certification, needed innovations, etc). She would like to address some short-term strategies and tactics for healthcare organizations needing to select and implement EHR solutions in the immediate future to optimize the usability of their chosen system. She would also address how the RECs and others might assist with goal.

Some of the questions that will be addressed are:

- How to add usability assessments to purchasing decisions and implementation processes?
- What is gained by including usability goals and practices: broader physician adoption, more meaningful use of key functions, and more consistent collection of data for outcomes and quality measures?
- How RECs and others can assist in this effort?

Methods of Measuring Usability

Charles Friedman, Ph.D.,

Chief Scientific Officer

Office of the National Coordinator for Health IT

Dr. Friedman will introduce a spectrum of methods that can be used to assess usability. One end of the spectrum, the qualitative end, will be anchored by "connoisseurship" approaches rooted in methods of formal criticism. The other end of the spectrum, the quantitative end, will be anchored in laboratory methods rooted in experimental psychology. The goal is to promote recognition of the full range of methods that are possible and illuminate the strengths and weaknesses of each.

Health IT Design and Usability: Myths and Realities

Ben-Tzion Karsh, Ph.D.,

Associate Professor, Industrial and Systems Engineering,

University of Wisconsin-Madison

This brief talk will address 4 myths about Health IT usability: (1) Usability is only affected by software design. (2) Making software screens and layouts simple and consistent leads to usability, (3) data dense displays lead to cognitive overload or simple, Google-style displays are what we need, (4) health IT should integrate into clinical workflow.

Evidence-Based Usability Practice

Kai Zheng, Ph.D.,

Assistant Professor

Information Systems and Health Informatics

The University of Michigan

Dr. Zheng will focus on "evidence-based usability practice." In software engineering, there are things called design patterns (or interaction patterns when it comes to User Interface (UI) design and software usability) describing common, best-known solutions to recurring problems. In medicine, obviously we have evidence-based medicine which is based on a similar principle.

He would like to propose an idea of building a national library of "usable Health IT designs" that documents common Health IT use scenarios and current best-known designs for accommodating each of the scenarios---similar to the Agency for Healthcare Research and Quality (AHRQ's) national clinical guideline clearinghouse. Detail can be figured out later with respect to what is "best design," how we test them to make sure no alternative competing designs would perform better, who will contribute to the library, how it's going to be maintained, etc. He thinks this is something that may generate considerable interests and sustainable long-term impact. It could work better than trying to come up with some usability requirement/evaluation check-list, which tells what needs to be done but not quite much about how to do it.

The library may benefit from using the web 2.0 approach by inviting practicing clinicians to comment on the designs, provide improvement suggestions, and what's more interesting: submit "bad" designs that they currently suffer from. This would in effect create some negative incentives forcing vendors to improve the usability of their software products (and to readily adopt the recommended design provided in the library agreed upon by majority user votes). This could generate some really interesting dynamics. It can also help the library respond to innovations in the IT industry (e.g., iPad) more quickly as compared to a usability standard; the latter may become outdated at a faster speed than we may anticipate (large displays, tablet PCs, etc., all became popular only within the past 10 years; who knows what may happen in the next decade).

Methods of Measuring Usability

Scott Lind

Director, User Experience, Soarian

Siemens Healthcare

As attention to usability gains prominence in the discussion and evaluation of Electronic Health Records (EHRs), some have advocated for a single usability metric. A recent Agency for Healthcare Research and Quality (AHRQ) paper recommended designing certification programs for usability. This short talk will look at some of the broad issues in attempting to define a single, overarching usability metric that is both objective and meaningful for large EHR applications.

Impacting Usability with Appropriate User-Based Research

Janey Barnes, Ph.D.,

Human Factors Specialist

User-View, Inc.

Specific research methods are appropriate based on the research question at hand. Likewise, specific research methods are inappropriate based on the research question at hand. Dr. Barnes will discuss selecting the appropriate user-based research method based on the research and design questions for different phases of the product lifecycle. She will give examples of positive impacts to the product when appropriate research methods and measures are applied. Finally, she will discuss how matching research methods to the product lifecycle are key to the development of a Usability Framework.

Usability Testing at CCHIT

Alisa Ray

Executive Director

Certification Commission for Healthcare Information Technology (CCHIT)

The Certification Commission for Health Information Technology (CCHIT®) initiated simple, practical usability testing for ambulatory electronic health records in its independently developed CCHIT Certified® 2011 program, launched in October 2009. This first version of usability testing was developed following research and consultation with experts in the field of software usability; it is described in a Usability Testing Guide on CCHIT's Web site. To date, about 20 products have been tested in this new program and more are currently scheduled for testing.

Accessibility and Health IT

David Baquis

Accessibility Specialist

U.S. Access Board

The combination of funds available to healthcare organizations for purchasing new health systems technology, along with the release of new Department of Health and Human Service (HHS) Health IT standards, provides a wonderful opportunity to impact the development of a new nationwide IT infrastructure. Unfortunately, accessibility appears to be largely overlooked to date. If this is not addressed, there could be a cost involved when advocacy organizations file complaints. This short talk will discuss what accessibility means and will provide examples of barriers experienced by people with disabilities. The implementation of a strategic accessibility initiative will be recommended to ensure that Health IT is designed to be welcoming to all users.

Creating an Inclusive Infrastructure to Allow Affordable Access Across Technologies, Disabilities and Ages

Gregg Vanderheiden, Ph.D.,

Professor and Director, Trace R&D Center,

University of Wisconsin-Madison

Information technologies are becoming increasingly integral and integrated into health care at all levels. It is critical that they be accessible so that they do not present barriers to individuals with disabilities or those who are older. This includes not only consumers but people in all levels of healthcare including practitioners, data processing workers and public health information personnel. A key element in this solution is the accessibility guidelines, standards, and regulations that have been and are being developed. But in order for this to be practical and economical we need to ensure that accessibility tools are up to the task and that everyone has access to them. We currently have good accessibility tools for some disabilities. But we do not have good tools for all disabilities. And even where we have tools they are not affordable by all and we have only reached about 10 to 15 percent of those who need them. Proposed is a systematic way to build accessibility directly into the broadband infrastructure so that it can be available to anyone, anywhere, on any computer or computerized device they encounter. Further through a combination of shared network services, common components, and increased awareness and outreach is possible to increase the market penetration, lower the costs, and create the more powerful tools that we will need to access the newer information technology being continually introduced into healthcare.

The SHARP Approach to Electronic Health Record (EHR) Usability

Jiajie Zhang, Ph.D.,

Dr. Doris L. Ross Professor & Associate Dean of Research

PI & Co-Director, National Center for Cognitive Informatics and Decision Making in Healthcare

University of Texas Health Science Center at Houston

This presentation will cover how the Office of the National Coordinator (ONC) funded SHARP project on Patient-Centered Cognitive Support plans to address the usability barriers to Electronic Health Record (EHR) adoption and meaningful use. Both short-term and long-term plans, approaches, and deliverables will be covered. Methodologies, tools, and products from this SHARP program will be summarized.

TeachEHR: Who's Training the Clinical Workforce

Juan Gilbert, Ph.D.,

Professor and Chair, Human Centered Computing Division

Clemson University

As Electronic Health Record (EHR) and Personal Health Record (PHR) systems have entered the clinical workforce, the academy is left behind. The recent rush to get EHRs into the workforce has left the academy standing still and the future clinical workforce is being trained in the absence of modern EHR and PHR technologies. How will the future clinical workforce be trained for EHR/PHR systems? What are the core competencies they should learn and who's going to teach them? Dr. Gilbert will discuss these tough questions and others that are being researched at Clemson University.

Usability is More than User Satisfaction: 10 Principles of EMR Usability

Jeffery Belden, M.D.,

Associate Professor of Clinical Family & Community Medicine

University of Missouri-Columbia

Usability is more than user satisfaction. Dr. Belden will review 10 Principles of Electronic Medical Record (EMR) Usability with copious visual examples, and then offer evaluation and testing methods for finished EMR products, and suggest ways to rate the EMRs.

Building a Technical Framework for Usability and Accessibility of Electronic Health Records (EHRs)

Lana Lowry

Human Factors Lead for Health Care IT

National Institute of Standards and Technology

A recent Agency for Healthcare Research and Quality (AHRQ) report on Electronic Health Record (EHR) vendor usability processes and practices identified the lack of common and EHR-specific standards for usability and accessibility of systems. NIST's role in meaningful use is to establish technical standards in usability and accessibility of EHRs. In this presentation, NIST will describe its efforts to support development of standards and test methods for these standards.

AHRQ Research Efforts to Assess and Improve the Usability of Electronic Health Records (EHRs)

Matthew Quinn, M.B.A.,

Special Expert, Health IT,

Center for Primary Care, Prevention, and Clinical Partnerships

Agency for Healthcare Research and Quality (AHRQ)

AHRQ's Health IT Portfolio is focused on understanding and improving the use of Electronic Health Records (EHRs) and other Health IT systems for improving the quality, efficiency and effectiveness of healthcare delivery. For over the past two years, AHRQ has established and built upon a research agenda around the role of usability and information design in achieving this goal. This presentation will describe AHRQ's research agenda and projects in this area.

Enhancing User Performance and Avoiding Safety Problems Through Analysis, Discovery, Prioritization and Design

Ron Kaye, M.A.,

Team Leader, Human Factors and Device Use-Safety Office of Device Evaluation

Center for Devices and Radiological Health, U.S. Food and Drug Administration

Further remarks on Mr. Kaye's part will stress the importance of involving users in the design process, evaluating realistic work processes and enhancing safety through designing the system in accordance with user needs and the requirements of the environments in which the system will be used.

Appendix E:
Acronyms Used in the Report

AHRQ   Agency for Healthcare Research and Quality
www.ahrq.gov

ARRA   American Recovery and Reinvestment Act
www.recovery.gov

BPMN   Business Process Modeling Notation
http://www.bpmn.org/

CCHIT   Certification Commission for Health Information Technology
www.cchit.org

CPOE   Computerized physician order entry

EHR   Electronic health record

EMR   Electronic medical record

EPR   Electronic patient record

FDA   Food and Drug Administration
www.fda.gov

HHS   U.S. Department of Health and Human Services
www.hhs.gov

HIMSS   Healthcare Information and Management Systems Society
www.himss.org

HIT   Health information technology

HITECH   Health Information Technology for Economic and Clinical Health
Act, 2009

ICDR   Interagency Committee on Disability Research
www.icdr.us

IT   Information technology

| ITL | Information Technology Laboratory |
| | www.nist.gov/itl/ |

| NIST | National Institute of Standards and Technology |
| | www.nist.gov |

| NPII | National Public Inclusive Infrastructure |
| | http://npii.org/ |

| ONC | Office of the National Coordinator for Health Information Technology |
| | http://healthit.hhs.gov |

| PHR | Personal health record |

| REC | Regional Extension Center |
| | ONC has funded 32 Health Information Technology Regional Extension Centers |

| RFP | Request for proposal |

SHARP	Strategic Health IT Advanced Research Projects
	(four projects funded by ONC)
	http://healthit.hhs.gov/portal/server.pt/
	community/healthit_hhs_gov__sharp_program/1806

| SMART | Substitutable Medical Applications, reusable technologies (one of the four SHARP projects) |

| SNOMED CT | Systematized Nomenclature of Medicine-Clinical Terms |
| | www.ihtsdo.org/snomed-ct/ |

| UFuRT | Unified Framework for EHR Usability |

| UI | User interface |

| UX | User experience |

| VA | U.S. Department of Veterans Affairs |
| | www.va.gov |

Appendix F:
References and Resources Cited by Speakers

Patel

Fernandopulle, R. and Patel, N. How the electronic health record did not measure up to the demands of our medical home practice. *Health Affairs* 2010 April 29(4):622-28.

Koppel

Jha, A. K. DesRoches, C. M. Campbell, E. G. et al. Uses of Electronic Health Records in U.S. Hospitals, *New England Journal of Medicine*, 360:1628-1638, April 16, 2009.

Werner

McDonnell, C. Werner, K. Wendel, L. *Electronic Health Record Usability: Vendor Practices and Perspectives.* AHRQ Publication No. 09(10)-0091-3-EF. May 2010.

Armijo, D. McDonnell, C. Werner, K. *Electronic Health Record Usability: Interface Design Considerations.* AHRQ Publication No. 09(10)-0091-2-EF. October 2009.

Armijo, D. McDonnell, C. Werner, K. *Electronic Health Record Usability: Evaluation and Use Case Framework.* AHRQ Publication No. 09(10)-0091-1-EF. October 2009.

All three reports are available at: Agency for Healthcare Research and Quality. Health Information Technology. http://healthit.ahrq.gov. (Matthew Quinn of AHRQ also referred to these reports in his talk.)

Boone and Grayson

Resources on usability from the HIMSS Usability Task Force are available at: HIMSS EHR Usability. http://www.himss.org/ASP/topics_FocusDynamic.asp?faid=358

Selecting an EMR for Your Practice: Evaluating Usability. HIMSS. August 9, 2010, available only to HIMSS members.

Karsh

O'Hara, J. M. Brown, W. S. Lewis, P. M. Persensky, J. J. *Human-System Interface Design Review Guidelines.* (NUREG-0700, Revision 2), Nuclear Regulatory Commission, May 2002. Available at: Nuclear Regulatory Commission. Document Collections. http://www.nrc.gov/reading-rm/doc-collections/nuregs/staff/sr0700/

Zheng

Alexander, C. Ishikawa, S. Silverstein, M. *A Pattern Language: Towns, Buildings, Construction.* Oxford: Oxford University Press, 1977.

Tidwell, J. *Designing Interfaces: Patterns for Effective Interaction Design.* Sevastopol, CA: O'Reilly Media. 2005.

U.S. Department of Health and Human Services. www.usability.gov

U.S. Department of Health and Human Services. *Research-Based Web Design and Usability Guidelines.* 2nd edition. 2006. Also available at http://usability.gov/guidelines/index.html (Also referred to by Jeffrey Belden.)

Air Force Guidelines: Smith, S. L. Mosier. J. N. *Guidelines For Designing User Interface Software.* Mitre Corporation, 1984.

Apple Guidelines: *need reference* (Also referred to by Dr. Belden)

Microsoft Health Common User Interface guidelines: *need reference* (Also referred to by Dr. Belden)

Zhang

International Standards Organization. *Software engineering – Software product Quality Requirements and Evaluation (SQuaRE) – Common Industry Format (CIF) for usability test reports.* ISO 25062. 2006.

Stead, W. Lin, H. (Eds.). Committee on Engaging the Computer Science Research Community in Health Care Informatics; National Research Council. *Computational Technology for Effective Health Care: Immediate Steps and Strategic Directions.* Washington, DC. National Academies Press. 2009.

Belden

(See references under Zhang that Dr. Belden also referred to.)

UI Design Patterns, http://ui-patterns.com/.